BETTER EACH DAY

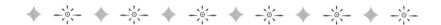

BETTER EACH DAY

365 Expert Tips for a Healthier, Happier You

BY JESSICA CASSITY

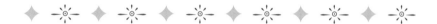

CHRONICLE BOOKS

SAN FRANCISCO

To my sister, Rebecca Cassity, and my "sister" Lisa Galaites.
You make all my days better!

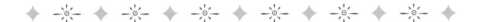

Library of Congress Cataloging-in-Publication Data
Cassity, Jessica.
  Better each day : 365 expert tips for a healthier,
happier you / Jessica Cassity.
    p. cm.
   ISBN 978-0-8118-7787-9 (pbk.)
   1. Health. I. Title.
RA776.5.C37 2011
613—dc22
                                          2010046891

Manufactured in China

Designed by Allison Weiner

10 9 8 7 6 5 4 3 2 1

Chronicle Books LLC
680 Second Street
San Francisco, California 94107
www.chroniclebooks.com

Introduction

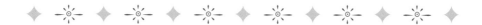

AS A HEALTH REPORTER FOR national publications including the *New York Times*, *Prevention*, and *Health*, I've spent most of my career asking hundreds of specialists about how to live better. And the scientists, yogis, psychologists, and other authorities whom I've consulted have always responded to my requests the same way: enthusiastically. They are eager to share their findings and observations, and hopeful that their work will find life outside of obscure peer-review journals and reach the general population, who can benefit most from their research. But once I get them talking, these experts often dole out too many kernels of wisdom to fit into a single article. So a few years ago, I found myself collecting notebooks full of these small but life-changing facts and incorporating them into my daily routine—slowly changing my eating habits, discovering the joys of cooking, deepening my yoga practice, and learning the best ways to unwind, one small step at a time. As my habits, outlook, and priorities began to shift, I realized that this information could change many more lives than just my own. With that in mind, I began working on *Better Each Day*.

The setup of this book is simple: each page covers one small change you can make in the pursuit of happiness, health, wisdom, and longevity. The tips cover a vast range of topics, from weight loss and anxiety reduction to how to be a better friend or why you should unplug from technology every now and then. All of the ideas are one-size-fits-all—that is, anyone can use them—but if you're like me, some will surely resonate with you more than others. Each of the 365 pages offers a fresh tidbit, so if a particular idea doesn't work for you or isn't what you're looking for at that moment, feel free to skip over it and keep reading. If you're looking for guidance on a particular topic, you can use the index to help you find relevant tips. There are no checklists or guidelines to follow. This collection of

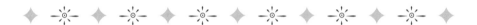

simple suggestions is for you to pick up and put down as you like.

While writing *Better Each Day*, I was reminded of just how many of these ideas have become second nature to me since discovering them. Take, for example, my conversation with Parker Palmer, PhD, the sociologist and community organizer who wrote *A Hidden Wholeness*: his insight led me to quit giving advice to friends quite so readily, and instead ask questions to help them find the answers on their own. Or one of the suggestions from Bonnie Taub-Dix, MA, RD, CDN, a dietician and author of *Read It Before You Eat It*, who recommends chopping a week's worth of veggies at once to make cooking over the following days a cinch. And there's Mark Liponis, MD, corporate medical director of Canyon Ranch health resorts, who got me to give up my midnight Blackberry habit for good—I had no idea that simply seeing bright light for a few seconds could cause my body to shift out of sleep mode.

And while those were unexpected benefits, some of the suggestions in here are ones I was actively seeking to help me find more balance and joy in my life. Using a tip from the book, one of the first changes I made was to stop ruminating—to cut out those long chats with friends where I overanalyzed the details of an event in the name of feeling better, and often ended up feeling worse. Amanda Rose, PhD, an associate professor in the University of Missouri department of psychological sciences, suggested imposing a short time limit on these talks—to vent once, then switch gears to keep from wallowing. I was surprised to see how easily I could circumvent anxiety by doing this. Now, when I start to worry about something, I try to head out for a nature walk in the park near my home: a number of studies referred to in this book show that just getting outside and into nature for five to twenty minutes can greatly improve your attitude and ease your mind.

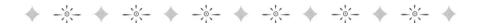

Many experts—from neuroscientists to yogis—put meditation on the top of their feel-better lists, but I honestly struggle to devote much time to sitting still. Instead, I learned to employ a different technique, one offered up by Linda Lantieri, a psychologist and author of *Building Emotional Intelligence: Techniques to Cultivate Inner Strength in Children*. I simply try to be present—and not get caught up in thought—while walking. By noticing my environment and the sensations in my body rather than running through my to-do list, I start to feel my mind calming down. Or I garden, which scientists and psychologists all agree will help bring peace and happiness into your life by quieting negative thoughts and drawing on your creativity and nurturing abilities.

That's the beauty of this book. It's a collection of ideas for you to take or leave at will—to try on and tailor to your life. Some suggestions may ring more true at a later time, and some never will, but all of them can be tested and tried until you decide which to keep and which to toss. And even if an idea doesn't work for you, it may be exactly what a friend needs to hear. Because all of the suggestions draw from the work of nearly two hundred top-notch experts in various fields, I have the utmost confidence in passing them along.

Writing this book has been an incredibly rewarding experience. Although I compiled the tips, it's the sources I spoke with who really gave wisdom and life to these pages, and I'm extremely grateful to them for being so generous with their time and ideas. Their research deserves recognition, and I am thrilled to share their findings with you.

I'm hopeful that just as this book has changed my life for the better, it will bring you the same gains in health, happiness, longevity, and wisdom.

OO1 Be the master of your own happiness

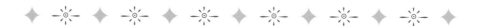

HOW MANY TIMES HAVE YOU uttered the phrase, "I'll be happy when . . . "? Whether it's getting a new job, finding the perfect partner, or losing a few more pounds, most of us are convinced that if we could just change one or two things in our lives, we could get our happiness back on track. Yet researchers have found that the most powerful influencer of our happiness is not what happens to us but how we choose to live our lives.

According to the Sustainable Happiness Model, put out by Sonja Lyubomirsky, PhD, professor of psychology at the University of California, Riverside, and author of *The How of Happiness: A Scientific Approach to Getting the Life You Want*, only 10 percent of your happiness is due to circumstance—the life events you have little or no control over, like your birthplace. Fifty percent is tied to genetics, which means that number is fixed. But that leaves a whopping 40 percent of your satisfaction dependent on intentional activity—the way you choose to use your time—which can include meditating, exercising, traveling, or whatever brings you the most joy.

Prepare a list of the things that make you feel good. Refer to this list to remind yourself what activities to engage in when times are tough. Whether it's cooking, volunteering, or working toward a physical goal, these are the things that can increase your mood infinitely, no matter what curveballs life throws at you.

OO2 Get a room with a view

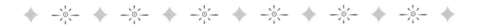

SPENDING TIME OUTSIDE CAN improve memory and instill a sense of calm. But what if you can't get into the outdoors? It turns out that viewing nature through a window can have a similarly restorative effect, according to research performed by Rachel Kaplan, PhD, professor of environment and behavior at the University of Michigan.

In a study conducted by Kaplan, residents of six low-rise apartment communities rated their satisfaction with the neighborhood and sense of well-being; those who had views of nature scored their quality of life higher than the participants who had views of buildings. While the specific settings varied, Kaplan points out that "nature," in this sense, needn't be a sprawling park or preserve. "Seeing a single tree can make a big difference," says Kaplan. "Nature comes in many forms, and having some is much better than having none."

Scientists suspect that viewing indoor plants, too, can have a strong positive effect on mood, and even more so upon the person who tends to them. So, to experience a greater sense of calm or satisfaction, adopt a houseplant or two. And, when you catch a glimpse of nature from your car, home, or office window, pause to take it in. You might find just the bit of hope, or calm, or vitality you need in a single tree or flower.

OO3 Be realistic about your resolutions

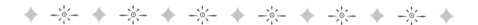

FITNESS GOALS CAN GET YOU motivated. But set expectations that are unrealistic—say, wanting to go from a decade of couch-potato mode to running a marathon in two weeks—and you'll soon give up your workout resolutions and end up back in the recliner. The trick to sticking with goals is to set ones that are challenging but attainable, says Gerald K. Endress, MS, fitness director of the Duke University Diet and Fitness Center.

To start, take baby steps to big goals. Focus on an appropriate goal for one month of training, like losing five pounds in four weeks, suggests Endress, or improving your energy levels. Then, make sure your fitness plan is realistic. You may commit to doing an hour of exercise six days a week, but if you can only guarantee that you'll hit the gym half of those days, set that as your goal. If you're able to go over that amount, celebrate! Finally, accept setbacks: if you aren't hitting your goals, decide if you've set your sights too high. If not, take some time to figure out why you're sabotaging your success.

OO4   Cure aches . . . with chocolate!

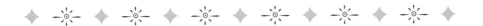

IF YOU'RE IN PAIN—WHETHER from a stubbed toe or a sore back—go ahead and pamper yourself. Relax, sleep, and, as new research recommends, eat chocolate! According to Paul L. Durham, PhD, director of the Center for Biomedical and Life Sciences at Missouri State University, indulging in some chocolate treats is a scientifically tested way to help the body heal from injuries and aches.

Durham, who has researched the effects of cocoa on healing, conducted a study in which animals that were fed cocoa, like that found in dark chocolate, had an improved response to injury. "Cocoa doesn't block normal inflammation, which is an important bodily response that prevents you from using an injured body part, but it keeps cells from over-reacting, which can ultimately lead to chronic pain." This response may be a better treatment than pain medications, says Durham, because chocolate doesn't mask the discomfort brought on by injury, which is a useful reminder to rest.

OO5 Ditch family-style meals to drop pounds

LOUD CONVERSATIONS AND heaping platters of food are two cornerstones of family-style dinners. Unfortunately, having all of that food so close at hand makes going back for seconds, or thirds, feel less like a choice than an inevitability.

To test this idea, scientists at Cornell University recently measured the amount of food consumed when eaters sat in front of or away from serving dishes. Not surprisingly, when the food was out of sight, it was also out of mind, though the degree to which serving style influenced eating was astounding. Without the temptation within arm's reach, participants ate 20 to 29 percent less than they did when the extra helpings were in front of them. To host family dinners that don't result in aching bellies, cut down on mindless munching by serving food away from the dinner table.

OO6 Authentic essential oils soothe stress

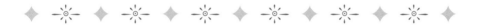

IF YOU'RE FEELING STRESSED, skip the lavender-scented candle. Sure, the flickering light and soothing fragrance can help you to create a more relaxing environment, but scent is just one part of aromatherapy, says Hope Gillerman, a holistic healer and creator of H. Gillerman Organics, a line of essential oil–based remedies and care products. While the smell of lavender may spark feelings of relaxation, the fragrance used in most candles is synthetic, and only the essential oil of lavender has a truly calming effect.

An essential oil is an extremely concentrated essence of a plant, and the particles are so small that when you sniff them, you actually inhale the essence, says Gillerman. Lavender in particular helps to naturally lower the body's levels of cortisol, a hormone released during times of stress. That's why the scent is so often associated with relaxation.

To unwind in the tub, Gillerman recommends you draw the bath and step into the tub, then turn the spigot back on and shake a few drops of lavender essential oil into the running water. This way you inhale the essence when it's at its strongest—right when it's exposed to air.

OO7 Look out for label loopholes

SCANNING INGREDIENTS CAN help you be a savvy shopper—and eater—but a lot of labels don't tell the full story of what's in your food. Food manufacturers know how to employ some sly maneuvers that make products look healthier than they actually are. Take a processed fatty food that supposedly has no trans-fats, for instance: "You may see zero grams trans-fats on the label, but if you look at the ingredients and see hydrogenated fats or partially hydrogenated fats on the list, the food still has trans-fats, albeit in trace amounts," says Bonnie Taub-Dix, MA, RD, CDN, author of *Read It Before You Eat It*, a book about food nutrition labels. These levels of trans-fats are low enough that the manufacturer does not have to legally acknowledge them on a label, but if a serving size is unrealistic—say, one helping equals two crackers, but you're more likely to eat a dozen—these trace amounts of trans-fats can add up fast.

OO8 Television viewing doesn't actually let you unwind

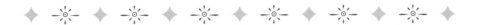

THE AVERAGE ADULT WATCHES more than four hours of television each day, according to the Nielsen ratings, largely in the name of "relaxation." But, the effects of TV are usually the exact opposite, says Marc Berman, PhD, a cognitive neuroscientist at the University of Michigan: "People think it's restful, because it's so easy to do—you just sit on the couch." But, rather than walking away refreshed, you could feel crankier and more tired with too much TV time.

"A lot of television is designed to keep you totally engaged," says Berman, who researches, among other things, the effect of different environments on memory and focus. So, while you may be hoping to give your mind a rest after a long day at work, you're simply engaging in a different activity that still requires all of your attention resources.

To actually unwind, consider an activity that really is restorative, one that allows your focus to soften. Meditation or exercise can help you ease your mind. Or, get outside for a walk and admire the view—being in nature has a restorative effect, and even looking at pictures of trees and other natural elements can be calming. "Nature gives you opportunities to reflect that other stimulating activities like watching TV don't," says Berman.

OO9 Be selfish to boost your benevolence

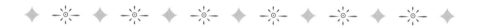

WHEN A FRIEND IS GOING through a rough time or a sibling asks for guidance, you're always there. It's true that helping others provides you with a feel-good surge, but over time, constant generosity can actually wear you out, and benevolent acts can become draining. The best way to really recharge is by taking time for yourself, says Linda Lantieri, director of The Inner Resilience Program, an organization focused on building emotional strength in school teachers. By taking a break, you'll keep compassion fatigue from setting in.

"Self-care—taking the time to replenish your emotional resources—allows you to fine-tune your own instrument, the way you relate to the world," says Lantieri. "Your generosity can't come from an empty vessel." To refill your reserves, make time for the activities you enjoy, particularly ones that leave you feeling elevated and calm. Yoga and meditation work for some people, while others turn to gardening, cooking, or creative writing. "To be compassionate toward others, you need to be compassionate toward yourself first," says Lantieri. Give yourself the space to de-stress and recharge and you'll be better able to offer support.

O1O Skip the multivitamin in favor of supplements

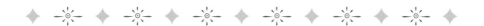

YOU MAY HAVE BEEN RAISED ON multivitamins, but new research suggests that these one-size-fits-all pills are actually a poor match for most people. If you already eat a healthy, balanced diet that includes a lot of fortified foods, you're likely better off taking supplements that contain only the specific nutrients you're lacking. If the foods you eat already satisfy your daily recommended values for vitamins such as B12, C, and A and nutrients like iron and folic acid, eating a multivitamin may actually tip your total intake well above levels that are considered safe, says Diane L. McKay, PhD, a scientist at Tufts University's Antioxidants Research Laboratory.

"You should always strive to get all of your essential nutrients from a well-balanced diet containing plenty of whole foods including whole grains, fruits and vegetables, beans and legumes, nuts and seeds, low-fat dairy products, fish, poultry or lean meats, and unsaturated oils," says McKay. Multivitamins, which contain a dozen or more types of vitamins and nutrients are best for people who are not getting an adequate diet, and or are at certain life stages that call for an increase in more than one specific nutrient. "People on a restricted diet including vegetarians, those who are lactose intolerant, or on a low-calorie diet, might consider taking a multivitamin to ensure they are getting an adequate amount of the essential nutrients for which they might fall short," suggests McKay. If you're only concerned about your intake of one nutrient, such as iron, seek out a supplement and skip the multivitamin.

O11   Keep your mind young

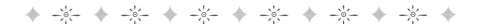

LEARNING NEW THINGS STIMU-lates cell function in the brain, keeping it healthy and youthful. For instance, when you travel to a new place and get to know your way around—say, memorizing your way from the hotel, to the cafe, to the Trevi fountain and back—you're actually helping your brain stay young by making new connections. According to Christine M. Gall, PhD, professor of neurobiology at the University of California, Irvine, tasks that require learning create actual growth in the ever-developing mind.

All sorts of learning activities can contribute to a healthy mind—textbook-based studying, active pursuits, and even mundane tasks. "Most things you pay attention to during the course of your day can count as learning," says Gall. "For example, recalling where you parked your car, or who you talked to in the morning requires learning and remembering information."

Learning new things is especially important as you age, because keeping the mind healthy over time requires increased maintenance. "The effects of learning through life will have more obvious benefits as one ages, when memory functions are not optimal," says Gall. Staying active and open to new challenges can help you stimulate and preserve this function. Sign up for Spanish lessons, tackle crossword puzzles, investigate a new hobby, or take a trip to a far-flung destination. Psychologists have linked activities like these with better recall of memories, too.

O12 Cut calories without sacrificing taste

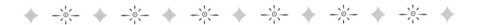

LIGHT COOKING SOUNDS GOOD in theory, but low-calorie foods often lack the flavor we crave. Luckily, there are simple ways to cut down on calories and fat without sacrificing taste, says Mona Laru, ADA, founder of Naked Nutrition, an eating, exercise, and wellness counseling service in the New York area. Substitute a high-fat ingredient with a healthier option to get the taste you want without the extra calories.

For example, rather than spreading mayonnaise on a sandwich, Laru suggests using Greek yogurt which has fewer calories, and more protein, and provides a tangy kick. To add even more flavor, mix wasabi, cumin, or lemongrass into the Greek yogurt. When baking, sub in applesauce for cooking oil or butter. "You certainly will need to do some trial and error, but the equivalents are typically the same," says Laru. Even main ingredients in dishes can be substituted: Rather than making fajitas with beef, try sautéeing slices of portobello mushroom with cumin, olive oil, and chili powder. You'll get more nutrients and a lot less fat.

Other tricks include eating a sandwich open-faced (using one slice of bread, not two), adding fresh-squeezed citrus juice to a salad dressing to cut down on the oil, or mixing your regular yogurt with low-fat Greek yogurt to retain flavor while enhancing the health effects. Also, look for lean meats instead of higher-fat cuts.

013 Improve your short-term memory

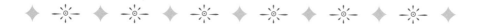

IF YOU FEEL LIKE YOUR MEMORY is fading fast, rethink the way you store and recall facts, phone numbers, dates, and more, says Marc Berman, PhD, a cognitive neuroscientist at the University of Michigan.

"One way to make short-term memory worse is interference," says Berman. "Old information you've learned can interfere with your ability to learn new information, and new information can interfere with your ability to recall old information." That's what happens when you try to remember too many similar things at once, such as four different phone numbers—they all get jumbled. To cut down on this confusion, create space between similar items when you're learning, like scheduling algebra class between French and Spanish lessons, says Berman, or taking a break when learning a new sport.

Of course, interference can also come from external sources: whether you're studying or concentrating on a conversation, your ability to retain information may be compromised if you're in a crowded coffee shop, in front of a television, or around other distractions. Though background diversions like music or game shows may make memorizing activities feel more "fun," your mind may wander, and your attention must go into overdrive to block out the extra stimuli.

O14 Ease back into exercise

WE'VE ALL TAKEN PERIODIC breaks from fitness. But if you've been inactive during the decade or two since your last touchdown, it's better not to jump right back into your old training routine. According to Gregory S. DiFelice, an orthopedic surgeon at New York City's Hospital for Special Surgery, the exercise program you used to follow may no longer be right for you. Once you enter your thirties and forties, chances are your body simply isn't as resilient as it used to be, DiFelice says. That means that the hill-running drill that used to constitute an average workout may now leave you with the muscle pulls, tendon tears, and sprains that DiFelice refers to as "Weekend Warrior Syndrome," named after people who exercise infrequently and push themselves beyond their abilities only to suffer from injuries. If it's been a while since you've exercised regularly, aim for at least three to five fitness workouts each week; just dial down the intensity and give yourself extra time to warm up, to reduce risk of injury.

O15 Use meditation to move on from mistakes

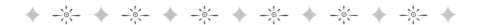

YOU'RE QUICK TO FORGIVE THE blunders of your friends and family, but what about yourself? If you make an error—be it something small, like forgetting to sign a school form for one of your kids, or a larger oversight, like saying something that hurts a friend—how long do you beat yourself up about it? Chances are, too long. According to Sharon Salzberg, author of *Real Happiness: Learning the Power of Meditation*, it doesn't do any good to feel bad and fixate on your mistakes. Instead, accept the situation, take a breath, and begin again.

The ability to forgive yourself comes from recognizing how you actually learn, Salzberg says. Do you learn and improve by blaming yourself for two hours for some minor error, or by seeing yourself more clearly and knowing to do things differently the next time? "There are lessons in the mistakes you make," says Salzberg, "but you only pick them up when you're able to forgive yourself."

To practice self-forgiveness, Salzberg recommends trying the lovingkindness style of meditation she teaches. With meditation, the goal is to let your thoughts move freely, but at a certain point your mind will likely wander off. When this happens, simply acknowledge that you've been distracted, but don't critique or judge yourself, says Salzberg. It may seem small, but it reinforces one of life's biggest lessons: move on from mistakes.

O16 Your Rx for a better doctor's appointment

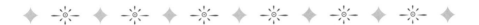

ACCORDING TO A RECENT REPORT, the average doctor's visit lasts eighteen minutes. That's not a lot of time, and you may have been rushed in and out of an appointment even more quickly, which can make it hard to share details about your health and get appropriate answers. The good news is that there are ways to maximize the minutes you do have with your doctor, says Ronald L. Hoffman, MD, a practicing physician and author of *How to Talk With Your Doctor*.

When visiting a new doctor, bring a concise, one-page written summary of your health, suggests Hoffman. If your physician has an easy-to-read document that lists your complete medical history, he or she will be able to easily reference your previous and current conditions and can better determine how a past ailment is affecting your present health. To avoid feeling rushed once you have your doctor's ear, prepare a list of specific questions—getting the answers you need will enhance the quality of the time spent with your physician.

To actually increase the amount of time you spend with your doctor, "Try to get the first or the last appointment of the day when doctors tend to feel less rushed," suggests Hoffman. And, show up on time. Late patients are often what throw off a doctor's schedule, and making your physician wait for you may result in an even shorter appointment.

017 Use yoga to create mental space

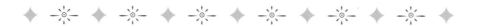

GIVING OTHERS SPACE IS ESSEN-tial for any relationship, but how much effort do you put into giving yourself space? According to Katie Malachuk, MBA, yoga teacher, life coach, and author, opening up physical and mental space plays a big role in keeping you healthy.

"Through yoga poses, we stretch, turn, twist, fold, bend, and even go upside down," says Malachuk. "This wrings us out, releases tension, and creates more room for digestion and for our vital organs to work. On a mental level, yoga teaches us to create space between ourselves and our thoughts."

Yoga is a form of moving meditation, a physical practice that requires you to focus on your body and breath. When mental chatter starts to creep into your practice—self-doubts, memories, to-do lists—you can simply return your focus to the body and breath to create distance between yourself and these habitual thoughts. Yoga's effectiveness lies in this repeated realignment to the present moment, says Malachuk. With continued practice, you can learn to create this space between yourself and your thoughts off the mat as well.

O18 Store your vitamins and supplements safely

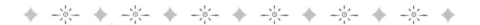

IF YOU KEEP YOUR VITAMINS IN a kitchen or bathroom cupboard, you may not be getting all the nutrients you think you are. Exposing vitamins to humidity can actually make the pills and tablets less effective, says Lisa Mauer, PhD, associate professor in Purdue University's Whistler Center for Carbohydrate Research. And some, such as vitamin C, can actually degrade completely in just a matter of days when stored incorrectly.

"Vitamins are best protected in dry, cool, dark locations," says Mauer, who recently studied the subject in her lab. If you store pills in a damp space, consider moving them elsewhere, like into your bedroom, where the humidity levels don't vary as widely. The original packaging for vitamins and pills is usually designed to protect contents from the elements, like light, but simply opening the bottle can allow moisture in; once the cap is closed, the humid air remains inside.

Some quality checks for vitamins can be done by sight: If you see any presence of moisture inside a container it's best to purchase a new supply. Also, beware of any brown spots that develop on the vitamins— this is often an indication that the pills have been exposed to moisture and their quality is waning. And, of course, keep an eye on the expiration date. Past-their-prime vitamins typically lose potency no matter how they're stored.

019 Regulate your coffee habit for more energy

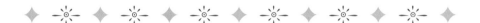

YOU KNOW THAT COFFEE provides a mid-morning distraction and an extra jolt of energy when you're feeling a little sluggish. But if you don't drink coffee every day, you may be better off cutting it out entirely. According to Peter Rogers, PhD, head of the department of experimental psychology at the University of Bristol, irregular coffee drinking can actually hinder your performance.

Rogers found that drinking coffee during the week and then consuming little or none on the weekend can cause feelings of tiredness and fatigue as well as headaches. To mitigate these effects, drink coffee every day, switch wholly to decaf blends, or drink a strong cup of joe only on the days you absolutely need it, such as during a long road trip. If you prefer tea or other caffeinated drinks, the same rules apply.

O20 Cheers, not jeers, go a long way

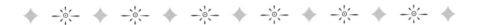

THE BEST COACHES INSPIRE YOU to do better, to push yourself beyond what you see as your limits, but coaching isn't limited to the playing field. "Many of the principles in coaching a sport are transferable to other relationships," says David E. Conroy, PhD, associate professor of kinesiology and human development and family studies at The Pennsylvania State University.

Encouraging words push a person to achieve, be it cheering a child on at a competition or coaxing a partner to open up and express him- or herself. "Warm and friendly encouragement works across contexts," says Conroy. In contrast, criticism and dominating behavior will undermine efforts to improve performance. Harsh words can even make a person perform worse rather than better.

Of course, the same principles hold true for yourself, says Conroy. Be gentle in your self-talk, and don't give yourself too hard a time if you make a mistake or don't accomplish something on your first try. A little TLC goes a long way.

021 Offset poor eating with OJ

BRUNCH IS DEFINITELY NOT
the healthiest meal of the week. With menu
staples including stacks of pancakes, plate-
size omelets, and extra helpings of bacon,
this feast takes the place of breakfast and
lunch, and probably *still* pushes your calorie,
fat, and carb intake over the edge. But if
you do indulge in the occasional Sunday
splurge, drinking orange juice can minimize
some of the negative health effects of a
big brunch. No, OJ won't burn through
all of the excess calories you consume, but
it can help ease the inflammation that
often accompanies eating unhealthy foods.
According to researchers at the University
of Buffalo, orange juice helps reduce the
number of free radicals in the blood after
high-fat and carb-heavy meals, and it can
also regulate insulin resistance. Of course,
this isn't an all-out free pass to eat whatever
you want—but to keep the occasional binge
from adversely affecting your health, a glass
of OJ can help.

022 Learn better after a brain break

IF A THOUGHT-PROVOKING movie, lecture, or book leaves your brain ready for a rest, go ahead and tune out for a little bit. Researchers have found that taking a mental break—like zoning out while you wash the dishes, or simply switching your thoughts to an easier topic—can actually help you retain any information you just learned. In a study recently conducted at New York University, people were asked to memorize pairs of images. Scientists measured brain activity while subjects viewed images and committed them to memory, and also a few minutes later, during a wakeful rest period. They found that absorbing information activated a certain spot in the brain, and in some cases, the brain became even more active during the rest period, which resulted in higher rates of retention. Daydreaming isn't a guaranteed path to better memory, but it's worth a try. In the middle of an intense study session, take a short break, then revisit the work and see how well you remember.

O23 Be realistic for best weight-loss results

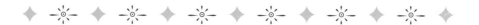

THE COVER OF A MAGAZINE boasts, "Lose 10 pounds in 2 weeks!" Before you jump in, ask yourself if what the article promises is realistic. The healthiest way to lose weight is with a combination of exercise and healthy diet, aiming to lose no more than a pound or two a week, says Heather Hausenblas, PhD, associate professor in the department of applied physiology and kinesiology at the University of Florida.

A doctor or a fitness trainer can help you to set realistic, motivating goals, and also come up with a plan to meet them. It's best to start small with weight-loss goals. Aim to drop a fraction of the weight you'd ultimately like to lose, and set a new goal only after your current goal is met. "If you set a big goal up front, like losing twenty-five pounds, you may lose motivation and get discouraged if it takes longer than you'd like, and that may cause you to ultimately give up," says Hausenblas. In the meantime, take headlines and fitness program promises with a grain of salt.

O24 Tiny tweaks will save the earth (and your money)

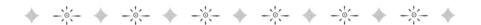

IF YOU'VE SWITCHED TO ENERGY efficient lightbulbs and carry your own bags to the grocery store, you're doing a great job of leading a more sustainable lifestyle. And more small steps like this can add up, says Jennifer Schwab, LEED AP, director of sustainability for Sierra Club Green Home, an organization that helps people green their living spaces. Before you purchase a more environmentally friendly car or plan a major home renovation, there are a lot of minor changes you can make right now, without a big investment, that will help you to lessen your impact on the earth.

Sealing your windows to prevent cold air from seeping in is one of the easiest and least expensive changes you can make to your home to curb energy use and costs, says Schwab. By running caulk along cracks and seams around windows, you'll create a barrier between the outdoors and the inside of your house, which means you won't have to use as much heat during the winter months. Regulating your water use is another easy fix: simply install low-flow showerheads and aerators to your shower and sink faucets to reduce the amount of water you use. Finding appliances that use fewer watts can also cut costs and energy. If your fridge or blender is on its last leg, look for a new one that has been labeled an energy-saving ENERGY STAR appliance.

O25 Eat mindfully, eat less

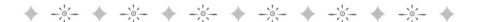

AN OPEN BAG OF POTATO CHIPS and a blaring TV are a sure recipe for overindulgence—distractions and mindless snacking go hand in hand. But you may fall into a similar trap even if you measure out a proper portion size, says Jeff Brunstrom, PhD, a behavioral nutrition researcher at the University of Bristol. If your brain is distracted from your food, it may forget to signal your body that you're full, which means you'll refill your plate even if your body doesn't need—or want—those extra calories.

According to Brunstrom, your mind subconsciously stores information about the food you're eating, then uses this data to determine when to eat next. But these mechanisms don't work if you aren't paying attention to the food you're chowing down. "In studies, we've shown that distracting people while they eat can impair the formation of these food memories, leading to more hunger and greater consumption of food at a subsequent meal," says Brunstrom. To fully absorb the food you eat—physically and mentally—get rid of all distractions at mealtime and pay attention to your plate.

O26　Give unconditional acceptance

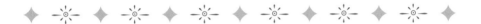

IF YOU'RE A "FIXER"—A PERSON who tries to help the people around you by showing them how to live up to their ultimate potential—you may think that your suggestions and encouragement are the best way to show that you care. But prompting a person to change or grow—even if you can see how necessary it is—is unlikely to produce much effect, and will often make the subject of your help feel scrutinized and judged, says Parker Palmer, PhD, author of *A Hidden Wholeness: The Journey Toward an Undivided Life.*

"When love and acceptance are contingent on a person doing something to make you happy, that actually decreases the likelihood that they'll do it," says Palmer. "Everyone needs someone who says, 'I love you as you are and I'll stand with you as you do whatever it is that you need to do, whatever it may be, including being just as you are.'" When you don't have stakes in a person's eventual outcome, he or she is more likely to trust you and to feel free to make changes—or not—with no one's interest but his or her own in mind. To take your ego out of the equation, remind yourself that we're all independent, imperfect beings, and the best support you can offer is to be present with another person without judgment, expectation, or an agenda in mind.

O27 Pay it forward

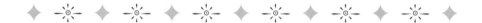

YOU'VE PROBABLY HEARD THE phrase "Pay it forward"—the idea that one good deed leads to another. It's a lovely concept, and one that recently has been backed up by science. In an anonymous, computer-based study, subjects were given money and the option to keep it or to share with a group. When a subject shared the money, a sort of domino effect occurred.

"We found there that generosity stemmed three degrees of separation," says study co-author James Fowler, PhD, professor at the University of California, San Diego and co-author of *Connected: The Surprising Power of Our Social Networks and How They Shape Our Lives*. When the money was given to a group of three anonymous people, those

three chose to pass it on to the next group of three they encountered, and the next groups did the same. The generosity only tapered off after twenty-seven people were touched by the giving gesture.

Acts of kindness needn't be large to make an impact on an individual or a network. And, anonymous deeds can inspire the desire to "pay it forward" just as much as an act that has a clear source. From washing your roommate's dishes, to adding money to a stranger's parking meter, to sponsoring a scholarship for a child in need, each good deed can inspire generosity far beyond your individual action.

O28 Eat rye to satisfy hunger all day long

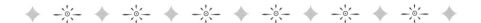

EATING RYE TOAST FOR BREAK-fast may be the easiest way to stop afternoon snacking. New research from Sweden reveals that rye bread helps increase feelings of fullness for up to eight hours. In the study, which was co-authored by Hanna Isaksson, a PhD candidate at the Swedish University of Agricultural Sciences, subjects were fed a breakfast of either rye toast or wheat toast with margarine and apricot marmalade. When satiety, hunger, and desire to eat were measured later in the morning, and hours later in the afternoon, eaters of the rye bread reported feeling less hungry and less interested in eating.

"The fact that satiety remained high even after a standardized lunch indicates that there are physiological effects that prolong digestion," says Isaksson. The high fiber content in rye bread is thought to be the key factor to this prolonged feeling of fullness, but Isaksson thinks that psychology may play into the results, too: she says that people expect dark breads to keep them full for longer than lighter-colored ones.

A more satisfying meal is hard to argue with, particularly if you're hoping to curb cravings. Similar results were found in breads containing varying amounts of rye, so test a few types to see which kind tastes best. If you're an oatmeal eater, rye porridge has been shown to have similar effects to rye toast, so it can be considered an appropriate alternative.

029 Skip meditation for music

IF YOU'RE FEELING STRESSED OUT, you might think your best bet is to reach for a recording of a guided meditation. But if you're hoping to listen away your troubles, you'll get better results from simply putting on your favorite tunes. According to a study recently published in the journal *Psychosomatic Medicine*, self-selected music relieves stress more effectively than relaxation tapes.

In the study, when participants listened to their own music, their physical symptoms of stress decreased just as they would have after a bout of exercise. Scientists think that by listening to something that actually led to positive emotions—rather than just relaxation—the test subjects were able to lower their stress reactions. The best news is that you can easily re-create the effect—just slide your favorite CD into the stereo or plug into your MP3 player, and let any tension melt away.

O30 Break a sweat for better sex

YOU ALREADY HAVE A HANDFUL of tricks to turn up the heat in the bedroom: soft music, candles, a bottle of bubbly. But now you can add another item to the list—your bicycle. According to researchers in Texas, aerobic activity like cycling can help women get in the mood. In one study, scientists measured women's level of arousal after watching two films in a row, one that was neutral and one that was erotic. On a separate occasion, the women pedaled on a stationary bike for thirty minutes before viewing the same films. Following the fitness blast, the women were more aroused overall and became aroused more quickly. Scientists think that the increased heart rate and blood flow of exercise may actually prime the body for sexual activity, so even if you don't like biking, try a brisk walk for the same results.

031 How to handle troubling thoughts

LIKE IT OR NOT, OUR MINDS
wander at will, and the more we focus on not
thinking about something, the more likely it
is that we'll conjure up those thoughts, says
Jon Abramowitz, PhD, professor and the
associate chair of the psychology department at The University of North Carolina at
Chapel Hill. The good news is there are ways
to ease your anxiety when your mind drifts
to places you wish it wouldn't.

For nagging thoughts, like worrying about
why your significant other hasn't called, try
distracting yourself. Call a friend, pick up a
book, or head out for a jog. And, try to put
your thoughts in perspective. "By learning to
identify when you're jumping to conclusions,
you can start to shut down those thoughts,"
says Abramowitz. "Look at the evidence
from real life. If your boyfriend doesn't call,
how likely is it that he wants to break up
with you? He may just be stuck in traffic
and out of battery power for his cell phone."

032 Make exercise a habit

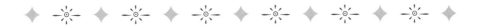

EXERCISE DOESN'T HAVE TO BE A grind. There are lots of ways to stay inspired and stick with a program, says James Maddux, PhD, professor of psychology at George Mason University.

When you first start exercising, it helps to focus on the big picture—such as an overall improvement in health. For many people, knowing that improved fitness reduces the risk of diabetes and cardiovascular disease is enough to get them out the door, says Maddux. Weight loss, too, is a big motivator for exercise. But keep your goals realistic: rather than working out to get the perfect body of the celebrity du jour, make your goal looking and feeling better than you do now.

If you start to lose steam, mini-motivations for each workout can help. "You may have a long-term goal of being fit, but daily goals—like being more relaxed, having an enhanced mood, and spending more time with your friends—will make you feel better immediately, which can help you to stick with fitness," says Maddux. For example, if you're going for a walk, invite your neighbor along and you'll turn your workout into a social call. Or, if you've been trapped inside your office all day, think about how great it will feel to get outside for a run, taking in the fresh air and getting that big boost of feel-good endorphins.

O33 Clean your house the homemade way

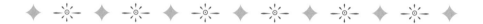

DIY HAS BECOME THE MO IN A lot of households these days, from growing your own herbs to crafting holiday cards by hand. Apply this spirit to your house-cleaning and you'll not only save money on expensive products, but also be sure that your scrubs and sprays contain no chemicals or toxins, says Cassidy Randall, program and outreach coordinator for Women's Voices for the Earth, a watchdog organization for the environment. You just need a handful of easy-to-find ingredients and an empty glass jar and spray bottle. Here are a couple of recipes to get you started:

ALL-PURPOSE SPRAY CLEANSER
(for countertops, kitchen floors, windows, and mirrors)

2 cups white distilled vinegar
2 cups water
20 to 30 or more drops of essential oil for fragrance (optional)

TIP: Warming in a glass jar in a microwave until barely hot will boost cleaning power for tough jobs.

CREAMY SOFT SCRUB
(for stoves, bathroom sinks, and toilets)

2 cups baking soda
½ cup liquid castile soap (find one that does not contain sodium lauryl [laureth] sulfate [SLS] or diethanolamine [DEA], which may have harmful side effects)
4 teaspoons vegetable glycerin (acts as a preservative)
5 drops antibacterial essential oil such as lavender, tea tree, rosemary, or any scent you prefer (optional)

TIP: Mix together and store in a sealed glass jar for up to two years. For exceptionally tough jobs, spray with vinegar, let sit, then follow with scrub.

034 Create good karma with generosity

HAVE YOU EVER WITNESSED A heartfelt thank-you or act of generosity, and been inspired to perform a good deed of your own? That's a natural reaction, according to the U.S.– and U.K.–based researchers who studied the power of the elevated feeling one gets from seeing others perform kind acts. In the study, people were asked to watch either a feel-good clip from television, a neutral clip, or a funny one. When it came time to fill out the questionnaire for the study, the researcher pretended to be unable to retrieve it from her computer. Participants were dismissed, then asked if they could fill out a survey for a different study, albeit a long and boring one. Those who had viewed the uplifting clip—in which mentors were lauded by students—spent almost twice as long filling out the form. This doesn't mean you should set out to do a nice thing just to have it come back to you, but the research does suggest that there's a lot of truth behind the phrase, "what goes around, comes around."

O35 Use past events to fuel future success

IF YOU HAVE A LONG LIST OF goals you'd like to attain but can't seem to muster the motivation or confidence to get started, here's one way to get a morale boost: write down all of your recent accomplishments. "When things are not going well, it's encouraging and comforting to look back at what you've achieved," says Ayelet Fishbach, PhD, professor of behavioral science and marketing at the University of Chicago Booth School of Business. When you're reminded of your drive, intelligence, and wherewithal to successfully pursue and accomplish goals, you'll have an easier time moving forward with the new projects and dreams on your list.

036 Outsmart the elliptical for real weight-loss results

YOU SWEAT IT OUT REGULARLY at the gym, so what gives when the cardio machine shows that you're burning a ton of calories, but the scale isn't in agreement? If you're not losing weight despite burning major calories on a cardio machine, the equipment you're using may be at fault, says Michele Olson, PhD, professor of exercise science at Auburn University at Montgomery.

"Unfortunately, the calorie-count mechanisms in treadmills and elliptical machines are often off by 20 to 30 percent," says Olson. So, if the readout says that you've cranked out 260 calories worth of exercise, a more accurate estimate could be 200 calories burned. "To even things out, I recommend doing 30 percent more than your target—so if your goal is to burn off 300 calories, aim to exercise off 390," says Olson. Even if your machine's calorie reading isn't that far off, increasing your workout time or effort should be enough to bump up your weight-loss results.

O37 Fill your plate like a pro

IF FAT GRAMS, NET CARBS, calorie counts, and vitamin requirements have your head spinning, one simple rule of thumb can make mealtime easier. According to Amanda Misrac, holistic health counselor and founder of Living Light Wellness in New York City, an ideal plate of food should look like a rainbow of colors.

"I like to start by filling half of my plate with leafy greens plus red, yellow, orange, and other colors of veggies and fruit," says Misrac. Split the remaining half of the plate in half again, filling one quarter of the dish with whole grains or starchy vegetables like a baked sweet potato, and the other with about 4 ounces of lean protein—around the size of a deck of cards. To round out your diet, add a small amount of good omega-3 fats to your plate, like olive oil in a salad dressing or a few slices of avocado.

038 Give hobbies a boost by practicing with friends

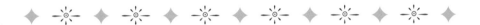

YOU MAY TYPICALLY PRACTICE your favorite hobbies solo. But research shows that sharing your top pastimes—like painting, dancing, and cooking—can actually help you to enjoy the activity even more. Case in point: Ann Skingley, PhD, senior researcher at the Sidney De Haan Research Centre for Arts and Health at Canterbury Christ Church University in New Zealand, has spent part of her career researching the mood-elevating effects of listening to music and singing, and she's found that the benefits of both activities are multiplied when they're done in a group setting.

Skingley works with an organization called the Silver Song Club, which offers older adults the opportunity to regularly come together and sing. Although her research has shown that listening to music and singing are both effective at boosting happiness, club members believe their improved sense of well-being also comes from getting together to share the activity. While Skingley only tested singing in the study, groups that center on other passions, like scrapbooking, reading, or cooking, can bring on similar boosts in mood. Plus, a number of studies show that feeling a sense of community and social support has a ton of other health benefits, including actually adding years to your life.

039 Exercise to beat cold season

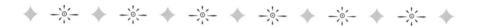

IF YOU CATCH COLD EASILY, think about investing in a pair of running shoes. No, a jog in the park won't necessarily cure a runny nose, but studies have shown a clear link between exercise and an enhanced immune system. In fact, some researchers report finding that people who work out regularly take half as many sick days as those who don't work out.

Aerobic exercise is your best bet for boosting immunity, says Mark Liponis, MD, corporate medical director of Canyon Ranch health resorts and author of *UltraLongevity*. Raising the heart rate increases the body's immune response and makes the body more proficient at killing bacteria and viruses. Some aerobic activities are more effective than others, according to recent research: Rhythmic sports, like swimming and rowing, provided a bigger boost than soccer or basketball, which tend to be more stop-and-go. Dancing and biking are two other good options, says Liponis. To get positive effects, aim for thirty minutes of heart-pumping exercise five days a week.

040 Use your mind-body connection to strengthen your resolve

IF YOU HAVE A HARD TIME flexing your willpower, try flexing your biceps instead. It turns out that clenching your muscles can actually help you to shore up the self-control you need to eat healthfully, commit to unpleasant tasks, and bypass calorie-loaded treats, among other good-for-you behaviors. In one recent study from the University of Chicago, researchers asked people to clench their muscles while drinking unsavory health drinks, while experiencing a painful situation, or when faced with temptation that was hard to turn down. When participants flexed—whether it was a finger, calf, or bicep that contracted—they all had stronger resolve, drinking more of the healthy beverage, bypassing the bad-for-you foods, and tolerating discomfort for longer. Use this tactic the next time you need a boost in willpower: simply make a fist and you'll skate through any situation with ease.

041 Make your workstation work for you

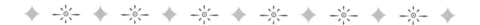

YOUR JOB MAY BE A REAL PAIN in the neck—literally. Regular computer usage has been associated with neck and shoulder pain, visual strain, and repetitive motion injuries like carpal tunnel syndrome. If you spend a lot of time sitting in front of a computer, it's important—and easy—to create a workstation that really works for you, says Karen Jacobs, EdD, OTR/L, a clinical professor of occupational therapy at Boston University.

Finding a chair that supports your back and allows your feet to rest on the floor is essential, says Jacobs. The keyboard and mouse are best arranged on the same level as one another, slightly lower than desk height, such as on an under-desk keyboard tray. Position your computer monitor on the desk about an arm's length away from you, raised to a level that allows you to read the top line of the screen without tilting or lifting your head. Don't forget to factor in screen glare, which can be an indirect cause of office aches: a compromised view may make you move closer to your monitor or sit with poor posture, so try to work with a light source placed at a 90-degree angle from your screen.

After you've established a comfortable workstation, keep aches at bay by changing your position often. Jacobs recommends taking frequent stretch breaks, such as making a prayer position with the hands to stretch the wrists, opening and closing the hands in fists, and leaning and twisting the torso to one side and the other. Simply standing up or taking a quick walk to the water cooler can also help you reset your body.

042

There's no harm in sleeping on an argument

YOU'VE HEARD THE SAYING, "Don't go to bed angry." But is there any weight to it? Will your chance to solve an argument float past if you don't reach an understanding in the here and now? Not necessarily, says Robert Gould, PhD, chair of the department of conflict resolution at Portland State University.

"Going to bed angry may affect your sleep," says Gould. "But, sometimes it's better to give the argument some processing time." By creating a bit of distance between yourself and the dispute, you may be able to better formulate your position and acknowledge what your sparring partner has said. However, it's not a good idea to put off issues indefinitely. According to Gould, "When an argument gets too hot, it's generally a good idea to let it cool down, but you shouldn't simply pretend it never happened."

043 Banish belly fat to fend off diabetes

HERE'S ANOTHER REASON TO lose that belly fat: scientists in Germany have found that a large waist circumference, even without a heightened body mass index, is a reliable indicator of risk for type 2 diabetes. To find out if you're at an unhealthy level, grab a tape measure and check your waist circumference, then move the tape down several inches and record your hip circumference. Calculate your waist-to-hip ratio (waist circumference divided by hip circumference). Women, if your waist-to-hip ratio is above 0.80, you're at moderate risk for type 2 diabetes; 0.85 and above is high risk. For men, the numbers are 0.96 and up for moderate risk, and anything over 1.0 for high risk. This high-risk ranking also ups your odds of acquiring other conditions as you age, such as cardiovascular disease and memory problems like dementia. To shrink belly fat, increase the amount of exercise you get, particularly cardiovascular activity, and stick to a sensible diet.

O44 Turn that frown upside down

HERE'S SOMETHING TO SMILE about: mounting research shows that people who smile a lot have more friends, are more engaged, and are happier, says Matthew Hertenstein, PhD, associate professor of psychology and head of DePauw University's Touch and Emotion Lab. That's because facial expressions are not just reflections of our internal state, they're also powerful signals that tell other people about who we are.

Take, for example, one of Hertenstein's recent studies: he examined old yearbook photos and was able to make a link between smile strength and relationship quality, determining that those with weaker smiles were actually five times more likely to go through a divorce. "I can't say that not smiling causes divorce," says Hertenstein, "but smiling is a reflection of an internal state, and by smiling we may attract other happy people."

O45 Another excuse to eat chocolate

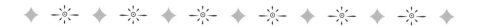

YOU MIGHT CONSIDER CHOCOLATE a miracle food just because of its taste. But chocolate and cocoa products really do provide a number of health benefits, from easing anxiety and lowering cholesterol to protecting the body from free radicals—and, according to recent research, chowing down on these wonder-sweets can also help reduce blood pressure.

New studies performed by Karin Ried, PhD, research fellow in the School of Population Health and Clinical Practice at The University of Adelaide, look at the health effects of flavanols, which are found naturally in cocoa. It's these natural compounds that appear to help regulate blood pressure. Dark chocolate typically contains the most cocoa, but check the label to be sure a bar has between 70 and 80 percent. At this stage of research, it's unclear just how much chocolate is enough to benefit your health, so be mindful of fat and calories when you're deciding whether to have a whole bar or just a bite.

If you don't have a sweet tooth, you're in luck: flavanols have been found in other foods such as grapes, red wine, and green tea, and other research from Ried shows that eating garlic may provide similar benefits.

046 Rekindle your relationship without changing a thing

IF YOUR RELATIONSHIP IS IN A rut, you could try to spice things up in the bedroom or book an exotic getaway. Or, according to research from The University of North Carolina at Chapel Hill, you could simply pay more attention to the thoughtful things your partner already does for you. In one recent study, couples recorded each moment they felt grateful for something their partner did, whether it was a small gesture like picking up the kids from soccer practice, or something larger, like preparing an elaborate meal. This increased awareness produced feelings of gratitude that often lasted for more than a day per act, and the couples felt more connected after paying closer attention to the generous things their partners did.

To get closer to your significant other, express gratitude for all the things—large and small—he or she does for you, and be sure to contribute your own acts of kindness, too.

O47 Talk yourself into a better mood

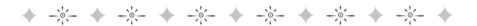

IT'S OKAY TO STICK WITH chitchat around the water cooler, but meaningful conversation is the best way to talk yourself into a better mood, according to new research. In a recent study that matched self-reported happiness ratings with conversation quality, people who had more substantive conversations felt happier than those who engaged primarily in small talk.

In the study, which was co-authored by Matthias R. Mehl, PhD, assistant professor in the University of Arizona's department of psychology, the conversations of ninety-seven undergrads were recorded over four days, then coded as either small talk or substantive. (Small talk was defined as trivial banter—like one-liners about the weather—while substantive conversation involved a sharing of ideas and information, like catching up with friends or discussing

opinions about current events.) Overall, higher well-being was reported by the people who talked the most and spent the least amount of time alone, period, but the happiest individuals engaged in a third less small talk and had twice as many meaningful conversations as the unhappiest people.

So how much deep conversation does it take to trigger an increased level of happiness? Researchers are hesitant to assign a value, but in a second study, Mehl found that "prescribing" just five extra fifteen-minute substantive conversations over the course of a week led participants to report feeling a bit happier. Rather than keep tally of your conversations, just look for opportunities to engage in a meaningful way. Your mood may get a boost, and whoever's at the other end of the conversation can benefit, too.

O48 Your friends can make you fit

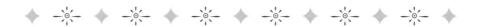

"ARE YOUR FRIENDS MAKING YOU fat?" That was a popular health headline a few years ago, spurred by the research of social networks and their influence, but according to one of the study's co-authors, James Fowler, PhD, professor at the University of California, San Diego, and co-author of *Connected: The Surprising Power of Our Social Networks and How They Shape Our Lives*, it isn't the full story.

"When the paper first came out, there was a pretty strong reaction," recalls Fowler. People thought that they needed to ditch unhealthy friends for fear of acquiring their habits, but researchers actually found the opposite to be true—rather than drop an unhealthy pal, the best way to stay healthy is to help your friend adopt healthier behavior. "We didn't find any evidence that the effects work differently for gaining weight than losing weight," says Fowler. Just as unhealthy behavior can rub off, so can a more positive lifestyle, whether it's adding more exercise or drinking less.

When you want to influence your friend to change, getting that friend on board isn't the most important step. Instead, change your habits and ask another friend to also adopt the plan—that way your pal is surrounded with good behavior. So don't just ask one friend to go jogging; ask a friend of that person along, too, and you'll all have a better chance of sticking with it. "If your friend is able to make gains and hold onto them, they'll rub off on you," says Fowler.

049 Soothe stress naturally with jasmine

YOU'VE HEARD THAT TAKING slow, deep breaths can ease anxiety, but you may not know that there's an easy way to maximize the effectiveness of your inhales and exhales: keep a jasmine plant or jasmine essential oil nearby. Researchers in Switzerland have found that the sweet-smelling flower has an effect on the mind that's in line with mood-stabilizing prescription drugs like Valium. The scientists are hopeful that jasmine fragrance will eventually take the place of the potentially addictive medications commonly used to treat depression, anxiety, and sleep disorders. When you need a bit of calm, sniff a bloom or sprinkle a few drops of jasmine essential oil on your skin or on a cotton pillow or tissue, and inhale the soothing effects.

050 Remember your big blessings to boost your happiness

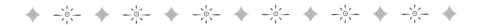

YOU'VE PROBABLY HEARD ABOUT gratitude journals—the notebooks where you write down all of the things, big and small, that you're thankful for. But recent research suggests that giving thanks for a specific kind of thing—the life-changing moments of your life—can be even more effective at increasing feelings of good fortune. In a study co-authored by Minkyung Koo, PhD, a research fellow and lecturer at the University of Illinois' College of Business, scientists found that looking at these major life events—even if they seemed small in the moment—deepened feelings of gratitude.

Instead of recounting the daily moments that make you feel grateful—such as your partner making you a cup of morning coffee—think about the instances that have sparked big changes in your life, such as meeting your mate, and reflect in particular on any fortuitous parts of the story. For example, if you met in a less than romantic setting, such as a bus stop, you can increase your overall feelings of luck and optimism if you start to look at the unlikely circumstances that brought you together (e.g., if one of you normally drove, but this one day you both decided to ride the bus). According to Koo, by homing in on the most meaningful experiences of your life, you'll bring about feelings of gratitude greater than those you get when recognizing everyday events.

O51 Use clear communication to resolve disagreements

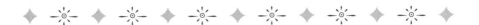

HAVE YOU EVER RESOLVED A conflict only to find out that you and the other person each walked away with a different understanding of the agreement that had been reached? That sort of situation happens all the time, says Susanne Conrad, a communications advisor who has helped companies around the world improve interpersonal and business relations. To take the confusion out of your communication, try this trick, suggests Conrad: simply repeat back to the person you're speaking with what you think they have said.

"Because we all have different interpretations of the same words, only when you try to explain what you think that person means will you know if you're both on the same page," says Conrad. And while this practice is useful for resolving conflict, it's also valuable for other everyday events, such as clarifying your responsibilities in a big project. When you repeat back your understanding of something, any differences of interpretation will be revealed. By bringing this to light in the moment, you'll be able to keep talking until you've reached an agreement not just in word, but also in thought.

052   Breathe easy

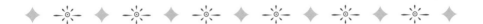

IF YOU'VE SPENT TIME RELAXING in a steam room, you may have noticed a menthol-like scent in the air. Spas and sports clubs often use eucalyptus essential oil to clean these dark and damp rooms—the oil is antibacterial, antiviral, and antifungal, not to mention more soothing to smell than a chemical-based cleanser. But the oil aids breathing, too, and helps energize tired bodies and minds, says Hope Gillerman, a holistic healer and creator of a line of essential oil–based remedies and care products.

To ease congestion, create your own formula for use in the shower or steam room, suggests Gillerman. Simply dilute ½ teaspoon of eucalyptus essential oil—found at most health food stores and some drugstores—in a small bottle of unscented body oil, and blend. Spread the formula on your chest and shoulders just before entering the shower or steam room. The heat, steam, and water will mix with the essential oil to create a vapor primed for inhalation. Keep this remedy handy during cold and flu season, or whenever you need an extra bit of energy.

053 Be smart about buffet-style eating

IF YOU TAKE THE PHRASE "ALL you can eat" a little too seriously, there are some simple strategies to minimize damage to your diet next time you're faced with a buffet table. According to researchers at Cornell University, buffet guests with lower body mass indexes (BMIs) left more food on their plates and chewed their food for longer than those with higher BMIs. The lighter diners were also more likely to sit facing away from the food tables and place napkins in their laps while eating. In addition to using these tricks to beat temptation at the buffet, opt for smaller plates when dishing your food and browse the entire selection before serving yourself.

054 Learn to screen the faux green

IF YOU'RE SWITCHING TO "GREEN" goods, be wary of the claims you see on products in the beauty aisle, says Siobhan O'Connor, co-author of *No More Dirty Looks*, a book that examines the use of harmful and hazardous chemicals in the beauty industry. The label of your favorite lotion may now boast that it's "organic," "fresh," or "green," but because there isn't any regulation on the use of these buzzwords, the ingredients may not be as natural as manufacturers would like you to believe. To tell if a product is truly organic—which means that the ingredients have not been sourced or grown in a way that uses persistent chemical pesticides, which are harmful to your health and to the planet—look for the USDA Organic seal, says O'Connor. Only this logo—which is the same one that is used for food— validates that the product has passed strict governmental standards.

O55   Lift your mood with music

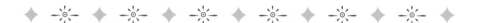

YOU KNOW THAT RUSH OF excitement you feel when your favorite song comes on the radio? Research now supports what you've long known to be true: listening to music you like can have a positive effect on your mood. That's the latest from Ann Skingley, PhD, senior researcher at the Sidney De Haan Research Centre for Arts and Health at Canterbury Christ Church University in New Zealand. In one of her studies, Skingley found that listening to music you find pleasing can reduce anxiety and make it easier to cope with trying situations, in addition to increasing overall happiness.

There's no need to let your happiness be subject to the whims of some DJ. To make use of this information on your own time, start collecting feel-good songs. These can be anything from instrumental concertos to Top 40 pop hits—just pay attention to what moves you in a good way. When you start feeling down or anxious, simply press "play" and wait for a brighter mood to set in.

056 Kill more germs with hand sanitizers

AS HAND-SANITIZING GELS HAVE gained popularity, hand washing has become largely water free, but if you're wary of how well these ethanol-based cleansers work, rest assured: a recent study from the University of Virginia School of Medicine found that using a hand sanitizer kills viruses more effectively than washing with soap and water. When researchers tested the effectiveness of each method in killing off rhinovirus, which is responsible for about a third of common colds, hand sanitizers that contained ethanol and organic acids did away with 80 percent of the germs while soap and water washed away just 31 percent. If you still prefer to wet your hands when you wash, steer clear of antibacterial soaps: in a separate study, these proved no more effective at killing germs than traditional soap and water, and scientists are afraid that the antibacterial formulas may help bacteria adapt to become resistant to common antibiotics, like amoxicillin.

057 Turn off technology to find tranquility

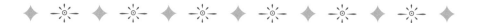

WHOM DO YOU SPEND MORE time with: your best friend or your Blackberry? Thought so. Technology allows you to be constantly connected, but that doesn't mean you have to stay available to everyone at all times. To give yourself time to recharge, get in the habit of setting aside time to literally unplug, says Linda Lantieri, director of The Inner Resilience Program, an organization focused on building emotional strength in school teachers. "I try not to turn on my computer at least one day a weekend," says Lantieri. "At the end of a stressful week, I need to shift out of work mode in order to be present during my time off." If taking a technology break isn't an option, set some boundaries for yourself, like not viewing work e-mails after 8 P.M., or avoiding social networking sites on the weekend. By limiting your online distractions, you'll be better able to engage with the friends and family who are physically—not virtually—with you, and make time for activities you enjoy, like reading or playing a sport, which help you recharge and beat burnout.

O58   Grow deeper relationships

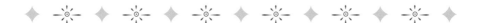

YOU'VE PROBABLY HAD SOME relationships in which you've felt completely comfortable, where both of you are able to be your true, zany, imperfect selves. What makes these relationships so different from other ones, where your conversations don't get as deep or you're afraid to put your real feelings into words? According to Parker Palmer, PhD, author of *A Hidden Wholeness: The Journey Toward an Undivided Life*, the cornerstone of a healthy, mutually beneficial relationship is a shared "safe space" between people, where both parties are able to speak freely and at the same time find their true selves.

This trust is built over time, and the goal is to create a relationship in which everyone feels heard, accepted, and not judged. Engaging in open-ended questions shows that you're interested in getting to know that other person without trying to change her, and may help her to explore herself a little deeper, too. To get "me" out of the way in these conversations, Palmer suggests asking yourself, "Is this a question I can ask without sitting here, thinking to myself, I know the right answer to this question, and I sure hope you'll give it to me?" By listening, but not judging, you'll engage in the type of below-the-surface exploration that can lead to a stronger connection and the feelings of acceptance that come from the best friendships.

O59   Get perspective on panic

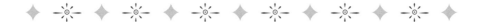

MOST OF US GET NERVOUS before a big presentation or a blind date, but if anxiety has made it hard for you to function—causing you to stumble over your words or making you feel numb or dizzy— it helps to address the situations that rattle your confidence. Luckily, says Michael Otto, PhD, professor of psychology at Boston University, and co-author of *Living with Bipolar Disorder: A Guide for Individuals and Families*, getting perspective on such a situation can be easy.

The first step is separating possibility from probability. Psychologists call this cognitive restructuring. Yes, it's possible that something will go wrong in a given situation, but how probable is it? "It's important to look at the situations that make you nervous and then reanalyze them," says Otto. "When you think something would be disastrous, with cognitive restructuring you analyze what could actually happen, how bad it is, and how probable it is."

Once you've addressed this worst-case scenario—realizing that it's unlikely to happen, and that if it does, it won't be as bad as you think—your panicked thoughts should soften, and you'll see the situation as less nerve-wracking. Your confidence will start to return, and after successfully navigating the situation that previously struck a nerve, your feelings of anxiety may disappear for good.

060 Dance your way to health and happiness

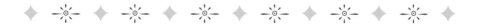

SPONTANEOUS DANCING MAY seem like something you do when you're happy, but dancing actually creates happiness. According to Jeremy Nobel, MD, MPH, a faculty member of the Harvard School of Public Health and founder and president of the Foundation for Art and Healing, dance is effective at treating and preventing mental and physical maladies.

Research suggests that engaging in the arts increases feelings of well-being, something that has been shown to help stave off afflictions like heart disease and treat conditions like stress, grief, and depression. And,

because dance in particular can increase physical fitness—and help you drop extra weight—it's what Nobel calls a two-for-one: an activity with benefits for both the mind and the body.

From ballet to ballroom to hip-hop, there's a style for everyone. Sign up for a class, dance along to an instructional DVD, or simply turn up the volume on your favorite playlist and get your groove on. Whether you're striving for a better body, a happier mind, a reduced risk of disease, or simply a fun way to kill time, a daily dose of dance may be just what you need.

061 Set better goals for a happier you

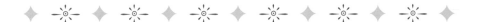

IDENTIFYING WHAT YOU WANT and the steps necessary to get there can add direction and meaning to your days and increase feelings of happiness. But some achievements can actually make you *less* happy, says Richard M. Ryan, PhD, professor of psychology, psychiatry, and education at the University of Rochester, so make sure you're setting the right kind of goals.

"We've found that people who are focused on materialism, image and popularity, or fame—things that we label "extrinsic values"—are more unhappy, and experience more negative physical symptoms and stress," says Ryan. "On the other hand,

people emphasizing community, relationships, and personal growth tend to be happier and feel healthier."

When you set goals, take the time to come up with creative ideas that align with your values and interests, such as learning a new trade or hiking in all of the national parks. According to Ryan, these will bring more positive feelings than goals like buying a new house or attending A-list parties, regardless of whether or not you achieve them. Of course, keeping balance in your life is important, so don't overwhelm yourself with a giant to-do list. Says Ryan, "make sure you also leave time to just *be*."

062 Trust your instincts about people

IF YOU'RE A TRUSTING PERSON, you may worry that someday someone will take advantage of your good nature and tendency to see the best in others. But rest easy—trust doesn't necessarily equal naïveté, according to research from the University of Toronto. In fact, in one study, people who believed others were generally honest and good-intentioned had an easier time spotting lies than those who were more skeptical. Scientists are unsure why trusting people are so skilled at detecting fabrications while wary individuals appear to be more gullible, but the study does suggest that those who are more inclined to trust are better at identifying trustworthy people. So if your gut tells you to trust someone, go with it.

O63 Don't skimp on sleep

YOU KNOW THE DRILL: YOU'VE
got a big work presentation or exam in the
morning, but you've waited until the last
moment to prepare, and now you must stay
up into the wee hours to get ready. Harmless
procrastination, right? Nope. Scientists at
the University of California, Berkeley, have
shown that sleep deprivation causes your
brain to function below its full potential.

In fact, a lack of sleep can deplete your
brain function enough that you're only able
to absorb 40 percent of the information you
try to take in. That means that when you're
tired, you need to study more than twice as
long as you would if you were well rested
to learn the same amount. Instead of pulling an all-nighter, grab a pillow: the same
researchers found that taking a nap as short
as ninety minutes can help refresh the brain
and bring back its learning potential.

064 Choose acupressure over Advil for headache relief

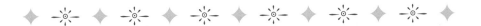

IF YOU'RE TIRED OF POPPING pills to ease headaches, acupressure offers a natural and medication-free way to get rid of pain fast. You may have already heard of the technique of squeezing the meaty part of your hand between your thumb and forefinger; this is one of the most commonly used acupressure points, says Venus Elyse, acupuncturist and founder of Integrative Healing in Fairfax, California. Simply pinch that tender area on either hand between your opposite thumb and forefinger and press for about two minutes, or until your headache subsides. This trick stimulates the pressure point called Large Intestine-4, and typically brings relief for traditional headaches.

If you're suffering from a sinus headache, you'll use a different pressure point for hands-on pain relief, says Elyse. To target this spot, called Urinary Bladder-2, firmly press the inner corners of your eyebrows with thumb and forefinger. You can rest your elbow on a desk or counter and lean into your hand to make this position easier to hold. The pressure needn't be intense, but you should feel a bit of an ache. After a couple of moments, your sinus pressure should start to lift, says Elyse. For best results, repeat either treatment about once an hour, holding for two to five minutes at a time.

065 Plan ahead to pump up for fitness

WORKOUT LOGS ARE SORT OF like food journals: the idea is that you write down every bit of exercise you do to keep an accurate tally and to get motivated to do more. Research shows that this type of accountability can help you stay motivated, but if spotty notes and blank pages aren't enough to get you back to the gym or out on the track, try this trick: Instead of using an exercise log to record the workout you just did, pen your training program the night before to give yourself an action plan. This way you'll have time to mentally prepare, pack your gym bag, and eliminate the chance that a last-minute excuse will undermine your efforts.

066 Wear red for romance

IT MAY SEEM CLICHÉD, BUT IF you're looking for love, you should wear something red. This is the color we tend to associate with romance, thanks to roses and hearts and Valentine's Day, but it actually triggers something much deeper and more primal, say researchers from the University of Rochester. Researchers have long been tracking animals' preference for red when courting, but only recently have they found similar preferences in people: in five different experiments, men rated females who wore red as more attractive and sexually desirable. Recent studies have also shown that women are drawn to men in red. So when you're picking out an outfit for a night on the town, take heed.

067 Stand up to improve your health

EVEN IF YOU EXERCISE EVERY day, spending the rest of your time sitting—at a desk, in your car, on the couch—can negate some of the positive effects of your fitness routine. In fact, in one recent study from the American Cancer Society, women who sat for more than six hours each day—less than a typical day at the office—had a 37 percent increased chance of dying from all causes, even if they regularly went to the gym. Research shows that sitting time can raise body mass index, blood pressure, and cholesterol, which may be what causes these increased health risks. To cut down on the time you spend sitting, try to add more activity in to your day. Consider biking or walking to work; if that's too far, park a couple of blocks away from the office to squeeze in a few extra minutes of movement. If you spend a majority of your time sitting at a desk, set an alarm on your computer to remind you to get up and walk around the office every twenty to sixty minutes. You can also increase your standing time by getting out of your chair each time the phone rings, using a smaller water glass that you need to refill more frequently, or relaying messages to co-workers by foot, not by e-mail.

068 Sharpen your mind with sports

YOU ALREADY JUGGLE DOZENS of responsibilities at once—so why not learn to *literally* juggle? New research from the University of Oxford shows that learning to juggle can increase brain connections—in one recent study, people who practiced the skill showed growth in the part of the mind responsible for hand-eye coordination and agility, skills that decline with age. Other activities that test the mind and body at the same time may have an equal payoff, so if juggling isn't your thing, try another sport that requires your complete attention, such as ping-pong, rock climbing, or partner dancing. According to the study, simply trying these sports provides the brain-boost benefit—the level of brain change was influenced by the amount of time spent juggling, not the level of mastery achieved.

069 Get a pet to prevent heart problems

PET LOVERS, HERE'S A REASON to give Fifi an extra-long tummy rub tonight: owning an animal is good for your health. This is the conclusion drawn from a number of studies, including one from the University of Minneapolis, which found that cat owners were up to a third less likely to suffer from a heart attack than non-cat owners. Scientists suspect that cats provide a buffer from stress, one of the leading causes of cardiovascular problems. While only cat owners were tracked in this study, researchers believe that other animals have the same effect on their companions. No pet? No problem. Simply volunteer your time at your local animal shelter to reap the health benefits of a four-legged friend.

070 Take small steps to stay organized

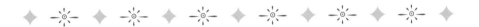

NO TIME TO GET ORGANIZED?
Just adjust your tasks to fit your schedule. While large projects—like reorganizing an entire room—can seem daunting, there's no need to tackle a big job all at once, says Emily Wilska, founder of The Organized Life, a professional organizing company based in San Francisco. There are a number of things you can do in just a few moments, and these small jobs add up to big improvement.

"Organization becomes much more accessible to people when they tackle mini-projects within a larger organizing project," says Wilska. For example, if the problem area in your home is the front hall, plan to focus on one small undertaking, such as opening and sorting mail. Once you've done one ten-minute task, you can call it a day or do more—either way, you've made progress.

You should also give up your picture-perfect idea of organization. According to Wilska, being organized doesn't necessarily mean that your home or office looks unlived in. It just means that you can quickly and easily find what you need, and that extra stuff isn't cluttering your space and your mind. To help an organized area stay tidy, and to avoid a gradual buildup of junk, set aside a little time each week to straighten up.

071 Silence your inner critic through meditation

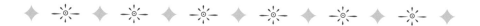

BEING HUMAN MEANS YOU HAVE to work through emotions you may not like. This is when compassion meditation may be most useful, says Sharon Salzberg, author of *Real Happiness: Learning the Power of Meditation*. Rather than eliminate painful thoughts, this practice allows you to reframe the way you think about yourself.

"If you feel an emotion come up that you don't like—anger, fear, or jealousy, for example—resist the temptation to label that feeling as bad, wrong, or weak," says Salzberg. "Instead, translate it from negative and judgmental terms and recognize it as a state of suffering or unhappiness." By no longer criticizing yourself for feeling what you do, you'll learn to be compassionate toward yourself.

Meditation is a way of developing this skill, says Salzberg: by practicing self-compassion during meditation, you'll be better able to draw upon it in real life. To start, set aside a certain amount of time each day to sit in silence. As you meditate, allow your thoughts to cross your mind and don't judge any of them. Instead, says Salzberg, "tell yourself, 'This isn't a bad thing to feel, this is a painful thing to feel.'" When you're more generous and accepting of yourself in these moments, you'll carry the kindness over to the rest of your life, too.

072 Get your house (and body) in tip-top shape

IF DUSTING AND MOPPING RATE higher on your to-do list than exercise, you may be in luck: a recent study found that how tidy a house is—or isn't—is a better indicator of the occupant's fitness level than the home's proximity to safe walking trails and sidewalks. Researchers are unsure if the extra physical activity involved with housework keeps the residents fit, or if the way people care for their homes is a reflection of the way they care for themselves, but the findings suggest that picking up a broom may be good for you in more ways than one. To maximize the calorie-burning potential of housekeeping, take small loads up and down the stairs so you must make multiple trips and integrate exercise into chores; for instance, do mini-squats or heel raises while washing dishes.

073 Think away your pain

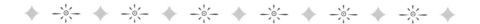

IF YOU HAVE CHRONIC PAIN, traditional medications aren't your only treatment option. In fact, painkillers may soon lose their spot as the most popular method of easing physical suffering, as more and more wellness professionals, including those at the Mayo Clinic's Pain Rehabilitation Center, use behavior therapy to help patients manage the condition.

According to research, distraction can provide a powerful form of pain management: simply shifting your attention away from discomforts can diminish your symptoms.

Imagining peaceful scenes has also proven effective at alleviating pain, though research hasn't established exactly which thoughts work best, says Chantal Berna, PhD, a researcher in the University of Oxford department of psychiatry.

Experiment with different techniques, such as listening to music, picking up a book, or reminiscing about a fun night out with friends. If these don't provide relief, consider hypnosis: this more intense form of treatment has also been shown to provide a great degree of pain relief, says Berna.

074 Take a break to refocus

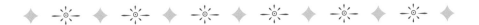

YOU SWITCH GEARS CONSTANTLY throughout your day, moving from one office task to another or from manager-mode to parent-mode, and often you've got to make the shift almost instantaneously. If these transitions aren't happening as seamlessly as you'd like, an intermediary activity could help, says Gabriela Corá, MD, MBA, founder of the Executive Health & Wealth Institute in Miami, Florida, and author of *Leading Under Pressure*.

"If you've been very focused on one activity, create a diversion when you start to feel burnt out or when it's time to transition to a new task, so you can come back with renewed energy," says Corá. Transitions can include having a meal, flipping through a magazine, catching up with a friend on the phone, hitting the gym, or simply walking around the block—anything that takes your focus away from what you were doing and allows you to regroup. "If you need to shift direction from one project to the next, I recommend transitions of at least twenty minutes," says Corá. "Any less time makes the switch more difficult."

075 Nix negativity to prevent health problems

A NEGATIVE ATTITUDE HARMS more than just your social life. It turns out how you think and act has as much influence on your health as what you eat or how frequently you exercise. In a recent study by the U.S. National Institute on Aging, more than five thousand people filled out a personality questionnaire in which they rated themselves in terms of agreeableness. The people who scored high in categories like skepticism, distrust, cynicism, self-centeredness, and arrogance were more likely to have hardening of the arteries when compared to the more agreeable folks. Based on these findings, the more negative a person is, the greater his or her risk for heart disease or stroke. If you tend to see the glass as half empty, exercise your optimism more frequently to protect your health.

076 Go green when you clean

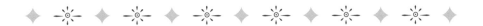

CHOOSING ORGANICALLY GROWN foods cuts down your exposure to chemicals, but the fight against health-harming toxins doesn't stop in your kitchen. Most likely, you use cleaning products that contain similarly unhealthy ingredients—but thankfully, it just takes a little know-how to determine which products need to be replaced and which are risk-free.

"Cleaning product companies aren't required to list the ingredients in their products, which makes it hard for consumers to stay away from chemicals they may be concerned about," says Cassidy Randall, program and outreach coordinator for Women's Voices for the Earth, a watchdog organization for the environment. However, some companies are beginning to list ingredients on their Web sites, so you can log on and search for products that don't contain toxins like allergens, ammonia, chlorine bleach, nano-silver, phthalates, synthetic musks, or triclocarbons, among others. These chemicals can irritate, over-disinfect, or cause a variety of hazardous side effects. Even if a product's label proclaims it to be "green" or "natural," it's worth investigating further: there's no government regulation of these terms, and what seems safe to a manufacturer may not measure up for you.

077 Nature can inspire more nurture

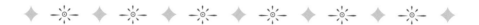

AS IF YOU NEEDED ANOTHER reason to visit the park, beach, or forest: recent research shows that spending time outdoors increases generosity. In one study, Richard M. Ryan, PhD, professor of psychology, psychiatry, and education at the University of Rochester, found that people who spent time in nature thought more about acting in the best interest of others, whereas people who spent a lot of time indoors were more focused on serving themselves. Scientists have yet to fully establish how the relationship between

giving and nature works, but Ryan says it's clear that nature puts us in touch with more positive and socially conscious sensibilities.

You may be tempted to take your boss for a walk to see if it results in your getting a raise, but it seems like this concept is better applied to yourself. So the next time you have a tough decision to make, head outside. You may better ensure that you make a fair choice, and you'll gain some newfound perspective: several studies have shown that nature walks can help you examine a situation in a new way.

078 Talk for health (and happiness)

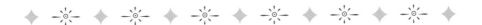

GOOD NEWS FOR CHRONIC chatterers: "People who talk more are more likely to be happier," says Matthias R. Mehl, PhD, assistant professor in the department of psychology at the University of Arizona.

Mehl studied the conversations of both men and women and found that on average, people speak about sixteen thousand words a day. (Yes, the notion that women talk more is a myth.) Of course, we all have our own degree of extroversion and openness, and various factors influence how much we talk or remain silent on a specific day, but overall, Mehl's research found that those who reported regular interactions rated their levels of happiness higher.

"The amount of talking a person does provides reliable information about that person's level of happiness," says Mehl. "Simply put, people who spend more time talking with others, by definition spend more time with others, and we know that being socially connected and integrated is an important factor for happiness."

The happiest individuals spent about 25 percent less time alone, and about 70 percent more time talking than the unhappiest people, based on self-reported levels of happiness. Certain careers, lifestyles, and hobbies can leave us more isolated— and less conversation-prone—than others, so if you find yourself missing the healthy effects of regular chatting, reach out to your friends, or join a group that will increase your social interactions.

079 To get fit, adjust your exercise attitude

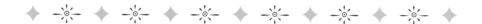

EVERYDAY ACTIVITY—LIKE TAKING the stairs instead of the elevator, or standing while talking on the phone—can burn up to 350 extra calories each day, according to research done at the Mayo Clinic. But if you don't have a good attitude about exercise in general, it may affect how much "non-exercise" activity you engage in, says David E. Conroy, PhD, associate professor of kinesiology and human development and family studies at The Pennsylvania State University.

In Conroy's recent research, he found that your implicit attitudes about physical activity—the beliefs you hold subconsciously—predict how much non-exercise physical activity you fit in. In one recent study, Conroy tracked people's reactions to photographs and words depicting physical

activity to see whether the response was "good" or "bad." Conroy found that the more strongly people subconsciously disliked physical activity, the fewer steps they took throughout the day.

To get yourself moving, find ways to change your conscious mindset. "Forming intentions to be active, setting goals related to activity, and making plans for how, when, or where to be active may be the 'easiest' way for people to increase their activity levels," says Conroy. Find an activity you like. Once you get used to that bit of extra exercise, everyday activities—like running errands by foot rather than car, or walking to a co-worker's desk rather than calling—may become second nature.

080 Meditate your way to patience and understanding

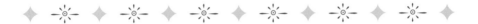

WHEN YOU'VE GOT A MILLION things buzzing through your mind, it's easy to get wrapped up in your own world and forget that everyone is interconnected. So while it may be your default mode to ignore strangers or be a bit dismissive when you're in a hurry, it's important to acknowledge people and treat them with compassion, says Sharon Salzberg, author of *Real Happiness: Learning the Power of Meditation*. Meditation can be the first step toward doing that.

"In one practice, we start with a repetition of certain phrases, like 'May I be kind, may I be peaceful,'" says Salzberg. Think the phrase, focusing on yourself first, then send the same blessing to someone you know—a person who's helped you, who is in trouble, or whom you feel a bit uneasy about. Continue to broaden the circle of people you think about, then eventually shift your thoughts to the whole world, sending the same message to everyone, everywhere, instructs Salzberg.

The practice is twofold: In and of itself, meditation is designed to teach us patience and acceptance. And, by reminding ourselves that everyone—those we know, and those we don't—deserves kindness and respect, we can learn to be more present in a given moment, more attentive to the people around us, and more understanding of the foibles inherent in all of us.

081 Keep your friendships healthy

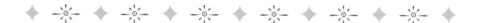

IF YOUR LIFE FEELS LIKE THE movie *Mean Girls*—complete with backstabbing, rumors, and all—this tip is for you. Relationship aggression—or trying to hurt others through their relationships or sense of connection to others—is a very real problem, says Amanda Rose, PhD, associate professor in the University of Missouri department of psychological sciences. And, while teenagers are notorious for these behaviors, we adults can act this way, too.

Rose says common behaviors include actively ignoring or excluding someone or spreading rumors. Basically, when a friend starts acting very contrary to how a friend should, you may have a relational aggressor on your hands.

It's hard to curb these behaviors in others—putting down another person often wins the aggressor attention so there's rarely incentive to stop. According to Rose, the best thing to do is to surround yourself with positive friendships and limit interaction with anyone who acts this way. If a friend starts to make you feel bad, consider if this is an intentional behavior. If it is, reevaluate your relationship.

082 Breathe deep to stay calm

WHEN EVERYDAY ANXIETIES creep into your life, it can be hard to stay calm, cool, and collected. Taking a few deep breaths may be just what you need to calm your mind and clear away tension, according to Elena Brower, certified Anusara yoga instructor and founder and co-owner of Virayoga, a studio in New York City.

First, bring your focus to the present—the position of your body, where you are, what you are feeling. From there, take a deep breath, sending air through your whole torso, lengthening the sides of your body, and filling yourself with a sense of your own worth, your own presence, says Brower. As you exhale, keep the space in your body but soften your skin and your eyes. Repeat this breathing pattern for as long as you need—until your heart stops racing or your palms are no longer sweating—and you'll be ready to tackle the situation at hand.

083 Find your feel-better foods

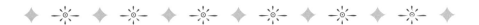

WHEN NUTRITIONISTS TALK about mood-boosting foods, they don't mean digging into a pint of Ben & Jerry's after a long, frustrating day. And though you may feel like eating something sugary—or salty, or savory—when you're cranky or tired, the best foods to balance your mood may not be the ones you crave. According to a study from the United Kingdom, when people were asked to cut out certain foods from their diets, they noticed a change in how they felt. The elimination of sugar, alcohol, caffeine, and—for some people—even chocolate led to fewer mood swings and less anxiety, while adding more vegetables, fruits, water, and omega-3-rich foods like fish helped people feel more balanced overall. Of course, our bodies all react differently to different nutrients and foods, so start keeping track of how you feel after eating certain snacks and meals, particularly when you're stressed. Use a notebook to record what you ate, then track your mood immediately after eating and for the next few hours. Keep experimenting until you've found foods that agree with your body and mind; start adding more of those to your diet while eliminating foods that leave you feeling down or unstable.

O84 Pare down your possessions painlessly

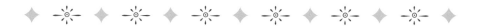

HAVE YOU EVER NOTICED THAT each time you tidy up a room, there's always an item or two without a home? Rather than stash it somewhere until the next time you clean, think about whether or not you really need it, suggests organization expert Emily Wilska.

Every object needs a place to live—otherwise, you'll never know where to find it or where to put it away. But when things go for a long time without naturally acquiring a designated spot, it's time to reconsider what the object is doing in your life, says Wilska. We often keep items that we think may be useful, but if we aren't actually using them, they just take up space.

To help you decide if it's time to toss, gift, donate, or recycle an item, tuck it away in a box for a month, suggests Wilska. If you don't think about it or need it, it's time to let go. Or, do reverse weeding, where you take everything out of a space, like a cramped drawer or closet, then decide what to put back in. By approaching your collections from the perspective of "what deserves to have a home" instead of "what I can get rid of," you'll be able to make more judicious decisions.

085 Stay sweet-smelling, safely

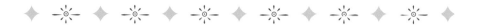

THE THOUGHT OF FORGOING antiperspirant may make you break out in a sweat, but there are real health reasons for considering a more natural approach to underarm care. "Sweating is one of your body's great ways of detoxifying naturally, and antiperspirant prevents some of that," says Siobhan O'Connor, co-author of the book *No More Dirty Looks*, which examines the use of harmful and hazardous chemicals in the beauty industry. "Additionally, antiperspirants also contain aluminum, and often triclosan, which have been linked to major health concerns."

But au naturel isn't the only alternative: plenty of natural deodorants have come onto the market in recent years. Simply test some out until you find one that works with your body chemistry, says O'Connor. Deodorants don't block your ability to sweat, so you may not stay as dry as you would with an antiperspirant, but they mask odor effectively and are usually chemical-free and less likely to stain your whites yellow. To make the transition easier, O'Connor suggests using an eighty-twenty rule in regard to use: "If you have a big meeting, a date, or a presentation, by all means use an antiperspirant. But for everyday situations, like going to work or hanging out on weekends, go with a natural deodorant. If you want, keep it close by so you can reapply on hot days."

086 Work out to up your willpower

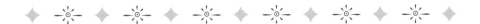

YOU ALWAYS HEAR THAT ANY weight-loss plan should combine exercise with a healthy diet—turns out this might be easier than it sounds, since the two elements seem to be a package deal. New research shows that sticking with a fitness plan increases your willpower for sticking with a sensible diet, too. During a recent study on exercise, weight loss, and behavior at the YMCA of Metropolitan Atlanta, women were put on a specific exercise regimen, but no strict diet—it was simply suggested that they eat more fruits and vegetables, and fewer processed foods. The subjects lost many pounds, but the calories they burned through physical activity accounted for just 10 percent of the total weight shed. The explanation: regular exercise led the women to report improvements in body image, mood, and confidence, says lead researcher Jim Annesi, PhD, which helped them better self-regulate when cravings struck. If you're having a hard time with your diet, start exercising. If you stick with a fitness plan, your eating habits may improve on their own.

087 Ease into projects for best results

YOU MAY THINK THAT UNWAVER-ing focus helps you out at the office, but immersing yourself completely in a task could be hindering your performance. If you throw yourself head-first into a work project, say researchers in Israel, you may not be as ready to handle unexpected events, like a new request that comes your way or a change in direction. In two recent studies, Israeli scientists found that the best way to ensure flexibility is to pace yourself. By approaching each task as a marathon, and not a sprint, you'll be able to keep reserves of energy stored away so that it's easier to maintain stamina, beat burnout, and be open to change.

088 Eat local for maximum health benefits

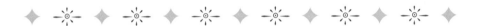

THE LOCAVORE FOOD MOVEMENT— eating foods that are grown near where you live—has gained traction over the last few years. It's good for the environment and good for you. While this concept of local, seasonal eating may seem new, it's one of the ancient principles of Ayurveda, an ancient form of holistic wellness.

According to Laura Plumb, teacher of Ayurvedic medicine and cofounder of the Deep Yoga School of Healing Arts in San Diego, food should be fresh, so that it retains its Prana, or life force, and transfers its living energy to you. The more local the food, the less it has to travel to reach you, and the fresher it will be. When you eat seasonally, locally grown food, you get the nutrients nature produces specifically for the season, says Plumb. For instance, in autumn we have lots of root vegetables that help build our strength and immunity for winter. Hit farmers' markets or research local growing conditions to find the best local and seasonal produce.

089 Clean house to clear your mind

IF YOU HAVE A HARD TIME forming thoughts in a cluttered workstation or messy home, you're not alone. Scientists in Italy recently conducted a study that found that a cluttered environment provided a lot of distractive stimuli, causing people to have a more difficult time focusing. Although the tests were actually in relation to fixing on a visual target, scientists believe that too much clutter can have the same effect on our thoughts, since it can be difficult to concentrate when our eyes and mind have more to roam over. To better regulate your attention, get organized. Commit to filing, folding, and otherwise organizing your possessions at least once a week in order to purge your surroundings, as well as your head, of unnecessary junk.

090 Fight disease with fungi

YOU KNOW MUSHROOMS MUST be good for you—they're veggies, after all. But their health-boosting benefits go above and beyond a lot of the other items in your crisper: Shiitakes help lower cholesterol and contain anticancer properties, and enokis can help strengthen the immune system. Now, new studies show that other (less exotic and less expensive) varieties also promote good health. White button and cremini mushrooms—which can easily be found in any supermarket—show significant health benefits, say researchers at Arizona State University. In a recent study of various types of mushrooms, Keith R. Martin, PhD, MTox, assistant professor in the school's college of nursing and health innovation, found that all types of mushrooms appear to be effective at reducing the risk of cardiovascular disease and hardening of the arteries. Try to add mushrooms to your menu a few times a week, incorporating several varieties into your diet for maximum health benefits.

091 Ditch the cell (even if it's hands-free) for driving safety

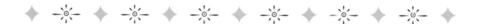

A NUMBER OF STATES ALLOW drivers to talk on cell phones while they're behind the wheel, so long as they use hands-free devices. Unfortunately, there's just no research to back up the safety of these laws, says David Strayer, PhD, professor of psychology at The University of Utah. Based on his research, and that of dozens of other scientists, using a headset isn't any safer than holding your phone while you talk. The problem with cell phone conversations isn't simply that you don't have both hands on the wheel—it's that the part of your brain that is essential to driving is distracted by your conversation.

This doesn't mean that all road trips must be silent: "When there's another adult passenger in the vehicle with you, you're actually safer than you would be driving alone," says Strayer. Even if you're engaged in discussion, the other person will likely keep his eyes on the road to point out distractions, and if conditions are poor, he'll know to keep quiet so you can focus. But start chatting with a far-flung friend, and your attention will no longer be in the car or on the road—it'll be on whatever topic you're talking about. Cell phone–related crash rates are comparable to drunk driving accidents, says Strayer, which should be enough to compel you to make your calls when you're out of the car.

092 Be honest about your workout routine—then improve it

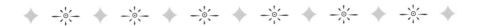

HOW CLOSELY DO YOUR EXERCISE intentions match the actual amount of time you spend working out? According to Heather Hausenblas, PhD, associate professor in the department of applied physiology and kinesiology at the University of Florida, most people—from the über-fit to the couch potatoes—tend to overestimate how much they exercise, so chances are that you, too, may think you're working out more than you actually are.

One way to get a clear sense of your workout habits is by recording how much you really do work out. Note the type, intensity, and duration of each workout; after two weeks, look back to gauge how much you're really exercising, then find new ways to fit in more fitness. Or, if your primary mode of activity is walking, invest in a pedometer. Wear the step-tracking gadget for a full week to see how many steps you average each day, then set new goals, aiming to top that number.

093 Invest in happiness

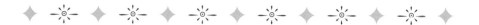

MONEY MAY NOT BUY HAPPINESS, but how you spend it might. That's the latest from Cornell University, where researchers found that the joy brought on by shopping usually peaks at the time of purchase, then steadily declines. However, experiential expenditures—like a weekend away or a kayaking lesson—create a boost in happiness that only increases over time.

Take, for example, two different purchases—a new couch or a vacation—says Thomas Gilovich, PhD, professor and chair of the psychology department at Cornell University and co-author of the study. If you need a new couch, taking a vacation may seem frivolous; the vacation will last a matter of days but the couch will be there for years. And yet, research shows that you quickly forget that it's a new couch, but the memories you create on a vacation live on and actually add to your sense of identity.

"You're a sum total of your experiences but you aren't a sum total of your possessions," says Gilovich. Investing in a vacation is one way to invest in happiness. Another, possibly even more fruitful, way to spend is to contribute money to your community to develop more local recreation options. "Investing your money, time, and energy in your surroundings is one of the easiest ways to ensure unlimited access to recreational experiences."

094

Sleep seven hours for the best benefits

YOU'VE PROBABLY READ THE long-established research showing that people who sleep five hours or less a night have a greater risk of acquiring several serious medical conditions. But new studies show that people who sleep nine hours or more in a single stretch have similar risks, including a higher occurrence of cardio-vascular disease. According to the findings from the West Virginia University School of Medicine, seven appears to be the magic number for sleep in regard to health—even resting for six or eight hours a night can lead to small increases in risk of heart disease. To slowly reset your nightly rhythm, gradually add or subtract to the minutes you doze.

095 Drink up to drop pounds

DRINK MORE WATER, LOSE MORE weight. This sounds too good to be true, but shedding pounds may really be this simple, according to a recent study from Virginia Tech. When people were asked to drink two eight-ounce glasses of water before meals for twelve weeks, they dropped an average of five pounds more than people who didn't add any extra water to their diets. The people who drank the extra H_2O ate an average of seventy-five to ninety fewer calories at each meal, so scientists suspect that the surplus water makes people feel full faster. The extra liquid may also result in the consumption of fewer sugary beverages, which is another way water could help you lose weight.

096 Think happy thoughts to get what you want

IF YOU'RE READY TO TAKE THE next step toward your future successes, be sure you've got a smile on your face. According to Ayelet Fishbach, PhD, professor of behavioral science and marketing at the University of Chicago Booth School of Business, a good mood can help you make headway toward achieving your goals. Based on her research, if you're happy, you tend to have less hesitation about starting new projects or making changes that lead toward your ultimate ambitions.

But cheerfulness does have its dark side: people with a more positive mood are also more likely to set aside their goals when temptation arises. So, let your happiness motivate you to start working toward a goal, but be sure that wandering attention doesn't steer you off course.

097 Make time to socialize over the stove

HOW OFTEN DO YOU COOK with a group of friends or family? According to Sarah Livia Szekely Brightwood, who runs Rancho La Puerta, a fitness spa and retreat in Mexico, and is the force behind the retreat's renowned garden and cooking school, cooking with friends and family brings great health benefits. But cooking in community is a tradition that has been lost over the last couple of generations. It's a tradition worth bringing back. "There's a reason that people gravitate toward the kitchen—it's the hearth, the heart of the home," says Brightwood. When you cook together, you not only get to enjoy sharing, you also get to laugh and work and play together as you prepare it. It builds a sense of community and brings joy to the table. Change up your next dinner party so that your gang gets together for cooking too, suggests Brightwood. You'll not only feed your belly, you'll nourish your spirit, too.

098 Sit up straight for instant self-assurance

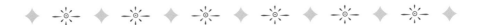

HERE'S A SURPRISING TWIST ON the notion that proper posture will make you appear poised and self-assured: sitting up straight actually builds confidence. That's one of the latest findings from Ohio State University, where Richard Petty, PhD, a distinguished university professor and chair of the school's department of psychology, researched the subject.

In his study, students were asked to either sit up straight or slouch while listing three negative or positive traits in relation to their aptitude for employment. Afterward, the students were surveyed on how well they thought they would do in future work settings. Regardless of the characteristics the students identified, the ones who sat with good posture were more likely to rate their abilities in line with what they listed. As in, the straighter they sat, the more strongly they believed what they wrote, rating themselves as either much more or much less employable than their slouching peers.

According to Petty, posture isn't the only thing that can enhance your belief in what you say or think. "Sitting up straighter, smiling, and nodding your head are all behaviors associated with positivity and confidence," says Petty. Do any of these as you share ideas (or even think them) and the people around you will think there's credence to what you say—and you'll believe it, too.

099 Walk off depression

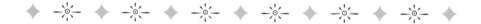

A STAGGERING 15 PERCENT OF Americans have suffered from at least one bout of depression. And while we all have negative thoughts on occasion, true depression—which is characterized as feeling down, experiencing a loss of interest and pleasure in daily activities, and having problems with appetite, sleep, or self-image—can occur when dwelling on negative thoughts becomes a cycle. Cognitive neuroscientist Marc Berman, PhD, says, "Through scans of brain activity, we've found that once negative information gets in the head of a depressed person, they have a hard time getting it out." Distractions and activities can temporarily relieve symptoms, but according to Berman, the thoughts usually come back when the task or activity is over. However, his research shows that rather than trying to shut out the thoughts, finding new ways to listen to them can help. The next time you're feeling down, head outside for a walk in a park. "Being outside helps you to reevaluate your problems in a softer setting," says Berman. Take in the sights and the sounds while allowing your mind to wander through the negative thoughts you're having, and you may actually help to lift them. If your symptoms don't lessen after about two weeks, contact your general physician.

100 Sneak exercise into your day

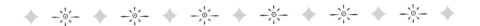

SPENDING A MAJORITY OF YOUR day sitting has been linked to obesity and an increased risk of disease, but a little bit of exercise throughout the day adds up! New studies show that adding even the smallest amount of activity can bring dramatic results, according to James Levine, MD, PhD, professor of medicine at the Mayo Clinic, who studies the number of calories you burn in everyday ways, like taking the stairs at work, or carrying groceries home from the store. He's found that people who incorporate activity into their everyday tasks—walking to a colleague's desk rather than e-mailing, parking at the back of a lot, and so forth—shed up to 350 extra calories a day. That's the equivalent of what you might burn in a forty-five-minute cycling class, without even breaking a sweat!

Invest in a pedometer and wear it for a day to see how much you usually walk. Then, set daily goals, aiming to up your step count to around ten thousand steps, or about five miles. You'll find it's easy to add more walking time to your days while at home, around the office, or running errands.

101 Strengthen relationships by learning to listen

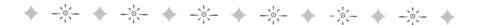

IF YOUR IDEA OF BEING SUPPORT-
ive is listening to a person's problems, then
detailing the right way to solve them, you
may actually be building a wall between you
and your friend. According to Parker Palmer,
PhD, author of *A Hidden Wholeness: The
Journey Toward an Undivided Life*, the mantra
for true friends should be "no fixing, no
saving, no advising, and no setting the other
person straight."

"When someone has a worried look or comes
to you with a problem, you'll probably invite
them to talk about it," says Palmer. But if
you listen for a few minutes, then start telling her what to do about it, your friend may
not feel heard or accepted. Instead, sit back

and practice what Palmer calls "deep listening"—when you suspend your need to be
a helper.

"A lot of us justify our existence by helping
other people, but often that advice shuts
the other person down," says Palmer. Let
your friends talk, and if they aren't finding
their own answers, ask questions that will
help them to explore their own feelings a
little deeper. "In creating safe space between
yourself and another person, your task is to
help them have a deeper and deeper conversation with themselves, not with you. What
you think they should do about it is more
about your ego than the needs of their soul."

102 Linger longer to eat less

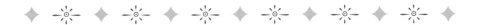

SLOWING DOWN THE PACE AT which you eat may help you lose weight. At least, that's what recent research from Greece suggests. Two groups ate the same serving size of ice cream; one group was asked to finish in five minutes, while the other group was instructed to eat the treat slowly over a thirty-minute period. Immediately after finishing, participants rated their level of fullness. Those who scarfed down the snack reported being less full than those who ate more slowly, even though both groups had consumed the same amount.

The lesson here: "If one eats slowly, hormones that signal feelings of fullness to the brain are increased, making it more likely that the person will stop eating sooner," says Alexander Kokkinos, MD, PhD, co-author of the study and lecturer of internal medicine at the Athens University Medical School. So, although the faster eaters eventually did feel full, they might not have sensed it until after dishing—and eating—another bowlful.

To linger longer over your next meal, limit your distractions so you can focus on the food. Turn off the TV, step away from your computer, and sit down with the intention of savoring your sustenance, whether you're alone or sharing the table with family. You can also split your meal into "courses" to change your eating speed: start with a salad, then dish up your main course. If you eat more slowly, and over a longer period of time, chances are you may not "need" to go back for seconds.

103 Something to smile about

"FAKE IT TILL YOU MAKE IT" CAN be applied to a number of scenarios but chances are you never thought it could help with happiness. While you may smile when you're happy, research indicates that smiling—even when you aren't happy—can automatically help boost your mood. "Not surprisingly, when we smile, we see ourselves as happier people," says Matthew Hertenstein, PhD, head of DePauw University's Touch and Emotion Lab. But there's a physical correlation, too: "There's strong evidence that when you smile your mood does improve," he says. "When the smile muscles in your face are contracted, you change your brain physiology and you feel good. It's not extremely powerful, but it does help over time, and it is good for you."

So, if you're happy, show it with a smile. And if you're not happy, smile anyway. That simple act alone may be enough to lift your mood.

104 For easy digestion, go gluten-free

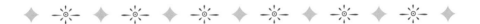

YOU MAY HAVE HEARD OF CELIAC disease, a condition that makes it difficult for the body to digest gluten, a protein found in wheat, barley, and rye. With diagnosis of the ailment on the rise—the American Gastroenterological Association estimates about one in one hundred people are afflicted—gluten-free diets and foods are becoming more mainstream. According to Ronald L. Hoffman, MD, a practicing physician and author of *How to Talk With Your Doctor,* even people who have not been formally diagnosed with gluten intolerance can benefit from eating gluten-free.

Because difficulties digesting gluten can be mild and hard to detect, take a week off from wheat (and barley and rye) to determine if you benefit from a gluten-free diet.

"A trial of gluten-elimination may reduce fatigue, bloating, digestive problems, joint pains, skin problems, and respiratory allergies," says Hoffman.

Avoiding wheat, barley, and rye isn't as difficult as it sounds. Many grocery stores have a gluten-free section. Pastas, breads, and crackers made from rice, corn, or potato starches and flours are widely available, and staples like meats, veggies, and fruits are still fine to consume. Make notes before, during, and after the week to track any changes in your health. If your reaction is significant, consult your doctor. If it's not, you may still find a few new favorite foods along the way. And, says Hoffman, eliminating starchy breads and pastas is a great way to lose weight.

105 Laughter is (literally) the best medicine

HERE'S ANOTHER REASON TO continue on the pursuit of happiness: whether you're suffering from a chronic condition or recovering from a recent procedure, keeping your spirits high can provide measurable pain relief. According to recent research, feeling down can actually enhance the unpleasantness of pain, says Chantal Berna, PhD, a researcher in the University of Oxford department of psychiatry.

In one of Berna's recent studies, when people listened to depressing music or had sad thoughts, they processed physical pain more emotionally and experienced it more intensely than they did without the negative stimuli. "Being in a sad state of mind and feeling low disables one's ability to regulate the negative emotions associated with feeling pain," says Berna. "When you're feeling down, pain has a greater impact." Luckily, other research has shown that the opposite is also true: in a separate study, when subjects' moods were lifted, the effects of pain were minimized.

106 With emotional lows come emotional highs

IF YOU'VE BEEN BURNED IN A relationship, you may be wary of getting back out there and playing the field. But, while your lowest moments may have happened because of a coupling gone wrong, researchers have found that our highest moments—the ones when we're happiest— happen within relationships, too. According to researchers at the University of Buffalo, interpersonal relationships—including romantic partnerships, friendships, and familial bonds—tend to inspire our most severe moods, both good and bad; they have an even greater effect than emotions brought on by solo accomplishments or disappointments, such as winning an award or losing a job. If you're feeling a little gun-shy after a bad breakup, give yourself the time you need to heal. But don't resign yourself to a life of solitude: while being alone may keep away some of the heartache, it'll also limit your joy.

107 Turn food scraps into fertile soil

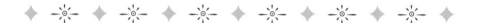

YOU MAY HAVE CONSIDERED composting your food waste—creating a bin that combines table scraps with yard waste, which slowly break down to become nutrient-rich soil—but have you actually jumped on the compost bandwagon? If you feel intimidated or overwhelmed by the prospect, don't be, says Jennifer Schwab, LEED AP, director of sustainability for Sierra Club Green Home, an organization that helps people to green their living spaces: composting is easy.

Start with a simple backyard composting bin, which can be found at most hardware stores. Simply set aside your food waste—everything except meats, fats, or dairy products can go into the bin. Add "green waste," fresh clippings of grass and other yard materials, along with "brown waste," which is made up of drier items, such as wood chips and cardboard. In your compost bin, aim for a ratio of about thirty parts brown waste to one part green waste so the new soil stays moist, but not wet. Turn the mixture regularly to keep it aerated, and you'll have your own super-rich soil to work with in about eight weeks.

108 Prevent type 2 diabetes the natural way

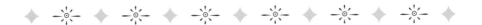

TYPE 2 DIABETES IS ON THE RISE, and because this condition and obesity are so closely related, the medical community has coined a new term, "diabesity." Diabetes means that you have excess sugar in your blood. Overweight people have a higher risk of developing diabetes, but thinner people with a high percentage of body fat are also susceptible. A simple blood test can determine your chances for developing the disease, so ask your doctor to screen you the next time you have an appointment.

If you're in danger of developing the condition, take action to reverse the trend. Studies show that weight loss through lifestyle changes can cut your risk, often as much or more than anti-diabetes drugs. "If you reduce your weight, you decrease inflammation, which can lead to an improved sensitivity to insulin," says Gregory G. Freund, MD, head of pathology at the University of Illinois at Urbana-Champaign's College of Medicine. "Instead of taking a drug, you're attacking the root of the problem.

"A significant proportion of type 2 diabetes is preventable," says Freund. Losing 7 percent of your body weight, implementing a fitness plan that includes cardiovascular activity and strength work, and adding more fruits and vegetables to your diet (while eliminating sugars and processed foods) have all been shown to increase insulin resistance, therefore reducing risk and incidence of the disease.

109 Tap into the benefits of massage (for free!)

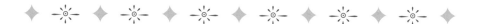

IF YOU'VE EVER LEFT A MASSAGE and felt as if a weight had been lifted off your shoulders—literally and metaphorically—there's good reason: new research shows that touch is good for the mind and body. "Studies show that massage reduces pain, increases immune function, enhances attentiveness to the world around us, and reduces depression," says Matthew Hertenstein, PhD, head of DePauw University's Touch and Emotion Lab.

Touch is one of the best ways you can invest in your life, says Hertenstein—and your investment needn't cost much. Physical connection, not technique, is key to stimulating the brain's reward center and triggering the positive effects of massage. Recruit your spouse, sister, or best friend to rub your sore spots. From stressed shoulders to overworked hands and feet, mild pressure is best at easing the muscles and the mind. Hertenstein suggests three fifteen-minute sessions each week, though he firmly believes even five minutes is better than none. And, offering to trade TLC sessions can sweeten the deal: research suggests massagers may experience many of the same positive benefits as massagees.

110 Go ahead, be a couch potato— as long as you bike or walk to work

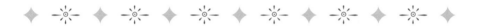

WATCHING TOO MUCH TELEVISION can be bad for your health, but there appears to be one way to get a free pass from its negative effects—by choosing an active way to commute to work.

In one recent study from Australia, more than fourteen thousand adults were surveyed on their health habits, including the time they spent watching TV, exercising, and biking or walking to and from work. There was a clear relationship between hours spent watching TV and body mass index (BMI), with more tube time leading to a higher BMI in both the inactive participants and those who reported exercising regularly. The eye-opening finding was that participants who either biked or walked to work saw no increase in BMI, regardless of the amount of television they watched. Scientists theorize that this difference between more formal exercise and active commuting exists because, while you must get to and from work five days a week, you can more easily blow off exercise on your own time.

To cut down on the negative health effects of TV time, consider active commuting. If your work is too far away to get to on your own two feet, find other ways of adding more activity to your everyday routine, like walking between stores when you're out shopping rather than driving.

111 Grow a garden to nurture your community

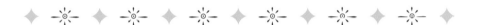

YOU'VE LOVINGLY DECORATED your house or apartment, and proudly call it home—but how connected do you feel to your neighborhood? If you want to increase your sense of belonging to a community, try planting a few flowers or herbs outside. One recent study from Denver shows that gardening—in your yard, and in particular, in a community plot—can boost your emotional connection to your neighborhood. Community involvement not only helps you to feel rooted, but also goes a long way toward improving neighborhoods by increasing contact and partnerships between neighbors, which can ultimately result in less crime and greater feelings of safety.

To shape your community, grab a shovel and trowel. Work in your yard, and if there's any common area that could be used for a garden—like a local community center or an empty lot—recruit a team to help you transform it into a more vibrant space. Tending plants is a proven mood booster on its own; by working together to spruce up your neighborhood, you'll benefit from the hands-on effect and the whole community will enjoy the drop in anxiety that can come from viewing and spending time in green spaces.

112 Ditch the routine to deepen relationships

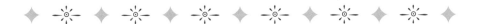

IF YOU WANT TO REVIVE AN OLD friendship, get closer to a colleague, or put the spark back in your marriage, break out of your normal routine. Shared experiences—particularly those that are unconventional, like rock climbing or a painting class—bring people closer together. "Doing novel or new things together can renew a relationship," says Thomas Gilovich, PhD, professor and chair of the Cornell University psychology department. The same is true of cementing new relationships—that's where the notion of unconventional corporate team-building activities comes from.

But don't feel like you need to go on a group safari through the Serengeti to connect with the people in your life. You'll get the same results with more low-key activities, like enrolling in a wine-tasting course with a friend or biking instead of driving to your favorite restaurant together. And don't stress if your activity choice turns out to be a dud: even bad times can strengthen connections. According to Gilovich, taking a date to a movie you both dislike will increase arousal and boost feelings of togetherness just as much as watching a movie you both love.

113

Join a team sport for optimal fitness and fun

HERE'S SOME MOTIVATION TO sign up for the company softball team: scientists at the University of Copenhagen found that women who participated in a team sport—in this case, soccer—were more likely to fit in regular exercise than runners who worked out solo. Though set training and game times may make team sports seem less convenient, the soccer players reported making it to the regularly scheduled sessions more frequently than the runners reported making it out for a jog. As a result, the team players' fitness levels trumped those of the runners. Researchers suspect that the camaraderie of the soccer team helped the players commit—psychologists say that while most people start exercising for health gains, many people stick with fitness because of the social support it provides. Case in point: at the end of the Copenhagen study, many of the runners joined the soccer teams, citing the desire to have fun with the other players as their top motivation to stay active!

114 Grocery shop for success

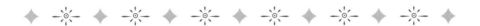

THE FIRST STEP TO EATING
healthier is shopping healthier. Whether
you're planning meals for an evening or a
week, a few simple guidelines can help you
to steer your cart toward more nutritious
choices, says Amanda Misrac, holistic
health counselor and founder of Living
Light Wellness in New York City.

"Whenever I take my clients on a grocery
store crawl, we start at the perimeter of the
store as opposed to the middle aisles," says
Misrac. At a typical market, you'll find vegetables and fruits lining the walls, plus dairy
products, meats, and fish, all of which have

high nutritional values. In the middle of the
store, which Misrac encourages her clients
to avoid, are the aisles stocked with highly
processed foods such as chips, crackers,
and cookies.

If your grocery list does take you to the
center of a store, look for whole foods. "A
rule of thumb that I always go by is the
fewer ingredients on the label, the better,"
says Misrac. You can also make allowances
for the aisle that houses spices and condi-
ments—these are typically healthy ways to
add flavor to the whole foods you pick up
on the outskirts of the store.

115 Know your antioxidants

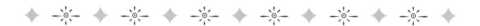

OVER THE LAST SEVERAL YEARS, antioxidants have become one of the health industry's hottest topics. But what are antioxidants, and why are they so important? "Antioxidants are compounds that can help prevent damage from free radicals," says Diane L. McKay, PhD, a scientist at Tufts University's Antioxidants Research Laboratory. In our bodies, free radicals—atoms, ions, or molecules that are highly reactive due to an unpaired electron—may play a part in conditions like cancer and heart disease.

Antioxidants are produced naturally in our bodies and found in many of the foods we eat. Vitamins C and E, selenium, and carotenoids like beta-carotene are a few of the most well-known antioxidants, and the richest sources of antioxidants in food are plants, says McKay. Whole grains, vegetables, fruits, beans and legumes, nuts and seeds, herbs and spices, teas, coffee, and red wine are all considered good sources of antioxidants. "There are thousands of different phytochemicals present in plant foods, and we are just beginning to understand the different ways in which they can function," she says. Studies show that people who regularly consume antioxidant-rich foods tend to have a lower risk of developing certain chronic diseases like cardiovascular disease, type 2 diabetes, and cancer.

116 Get a strong core in sixty seconds

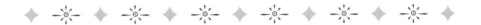

PILATES' RECENT RISE IN POPU-larity has brought even more attention to the importance of core work, which includes strengthening the muscles in your abs, back, hips, butt, and upper thighs. Whether you're lifting boxes or walking for fitness, strong core muscles will help you to move more efficiently and powerfully, says Kristin McGee, a yoga and Pilates instructor in New York City and creator of a number of mind-body fitness DVDs.

Crunches work a few layers of your ab muscles, but you'll need more challenging moves to build strength and tone your entire core. Try one of McGee's favorite exercises, the forearm plank: Start on your hands and knees, then bend at the elbows and place your forearms on the floor, making fists with either hand. Extend your right leg back on the floor and then your left leg, so that your body forms one straight line from heels to head, with your weight on your forearms and toes. Squeeze your legs together and feel your abs draw in and up, as though you're zipping up a tight pair of jeans. Build up to holding this pose for one minute.

117

Protect your skin from the inside out

ALONG WITH YOUR SUNBLOCK, shades, and big straw hat, research shows that a diet high in omega-3 fatty acids and antioxidants is a powerful weapon against skin damage brought on by UV rays. In a recent study, people who ate foods high in these nutrients—particularly red-pigmented carotenoids like those found in carrots, watermelon, and tomatoes—showed less skin damage than those who did not. The impetus for this study was fueled by the low rate of melanoma in Mediterranean countries, where people typically eat diets rich in omega-3 fatty acids and antioxidants. While the results by no means suggest that you'd be safe to go out into the sun without protection following a big Mediterranean-inspired meal, you can build up your body's natural defenses against the sun's rays by changing your diet.

118 Create a backyard retreat

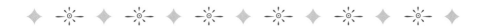

THERE'S NO REASON THAT ONE outdoor space can't accommodate a wide range of activities. It's simple to create a place to relax, work, and play in the outdoors, says landscape architect Sarah Livia Szekely Brightwood, who runs Rancho La Puerta, a fitness spa and retreat in Mexico. Just as a park is designed with different areas to suit various activities, your yard can contain several mini-spaces, becoming a place that will restore you, whatever your mood.

To start planning, don't just think of your yard as an empty slate. Instead, connect with the space and let it show you what's already there—notice the light patterns, the tree and shrub growth, and the soil type, suggests Brightwood. Then, think about how you'd like to move through the space, as if it were telling a story: each part of the garden is like a separate character, and the landscape plan should link one voice to another. Consider the types of environments you want in your yard—such as separate spots to be alone, to have company, and to work the land—then slowly build them. Maintaining a garden takes constant care, reminds Brightwood, so start small, then gradually expand.

119

Pick ginger to prevent post-gym pain

EXERCISE EXEMPLIFIES THE saying "no pain, no gain," but that doesn't mean you can't ease the discomfort a bit. When you push yourself during a workout, your muscle fibers tear only to rebuild stronger—that's why you may feel sore about twenty-four hours after a fitness session. To minimize the soreness brought on by exercising longer or harder than usual, follow this trick, recently discovered by University of Georgia researchers: regularly consume 2 grams, or about half a teaspoon, of ginger each day, and you'll likely experience around 25 percent less post-exercise soreness. To get your ginger fix, add freshly grated ginger to stir-frys, drinks like lemonade, or other dishes that could use a little kick.

120 Plan ahead to dine out healthy

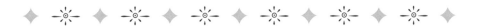

EATING OUT IS DIVINE, BUT IT'S easy to overindulge when faced with so many delicious choices. Having a plan in place can help you resist giving in to temptation, particularly if a glass of wine lowers your defenses, or a favorite creamy pasta dish is being offered as a special.

Eliminating the element of surprise is the easiest first step. "So many restaurants have menus online," says Bonnie Taub-Dix, MA, RD, CDN, and author of *Read It Before You Eat It*. "There's no reason you can't choose your food before sitting down." You may want to skip the entrees entirely if you're looking for a light night out. Choose

a salad and an appetizer instead of a main dish and you'll likely cut calories and get more nutrients, suggests Taub-Dix. Or, share an entree. Same goes for dessert—split a treat among everyone at the table or, better yet, order a decaf coffee, light on the cream and sugar.

Also, make sure you aren't famished before sitting down. "It's easier to make a rational decision if you aren't starving," says Taub-Dix. If you're on your way to a restaurant with a notorious wait, eat a cup of yogurt, a piece of fruit, or an energy bar about an hour and a half before you go.

121

Add variety to your workout

FOCUSING ON JUST ONE TYPE of exercise, like running or yoga, may not yield the best results. Studies show that doing the same exercises day after day isn't an effective way to train—as the workout becomes less challenging for your body, you'll burn fewer calories and make smaller strength gains. To get out of a rut without completely changing your routine, add a new activity to your regimen.

Cross-training, or doing a variety of workouts, gives you the chance to rest certain muscles while working others, says Kristin McGee, a yoga and Pilates instructor in New York City. And, incorporating new types of exercise helps beat boredom, one of the main reasons people stop working out. To get inspired, try a new class at the gym or look into outdoor activities like biking or hiking, suggests McGee. For best results, find a few favorite workouts, then add the occasional wild card to the mix to keep your body and mind fit and engaged.

122 Set goals to boost self-esteem

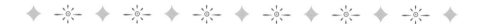

THERE'S A STRONG LINK BETWEEN low self-esteem and depression, but there's been much speculation about which condition comes first. Recent research by a team led by Ulrich Orth, PhD, a research professor in the University of Basel's department of psychology, has found that depression is often the result of low self-esteem, meaning that feeling down about yourself can develop into depression. Orth's theory is that people who aren't as confident may seek more reassurance from others, thereby opening themselves up to social rejection. Those with low self-esteem also tend to isolate themselves from others. Rumination, or the constant dwelling on one's problems, may be another factor.

Building self-esteem will lead to better mental health. There's no surefire way to increase your sense of self-worth, but one technique that often helps heighten confidence is to work toward a goal. For instance, if you're struggling with feelings of low self-esteem, learn a new cooking technique or stick to an exercise routine. As you master a new skill or commit to a healthy habit, you'll be left with a sense of accomplishment. Your self-esteem will benefit and your mood will get a lift.

123 Go outside for an instant sanity saver

IF YOU NEED A QUICK CRANKINESS cure, head outside. Just five minutes of activity in the outdoors can improve mood and reduce risk of mental illness, according to a recent report from the University of Essex. When the paper's authors reviewed ten studies on the effects of nature on various aspects of mental health, they found that even a few minutes of outdoor time increased subjects' happiness. To get the biggest boost in mood, researchers found that being active in the outdoors is best, so consider tossing a Frisbee or taking a walk. You'll feel better and increase your calorie burn.

124 Warm up for a better workout

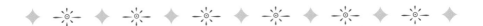

IF YOUR PRE-WORKOUT WARM-UP consists of bending over to tie your shoes, you may want to reconsider how you spend those pre-fitness moments: In a review of thirty-two studies, exercisers who warmed-up before a workout experienced a 4- to 12-percent boost in physical performance, such as being able to run harder or faster. According to Andrea Fradkin, PhD, co-author of the review and associate professor of exercise science at Bloomsburg University, warming up for about five minutes is all you need to take your performance up a notch.

Based on Fradkin's research, the best warm-ups are three-step routines fine-tuned to the demands of your activity. "First, a few moments of light aerobic exercise will increase the body temperature and get the blood and oxygen flowing." Walk, jog, or do another activity, like jumping jacks. Next, suggests Fradkin, stretch the muscles you'll be working so that you're able to easily move through your full range of motion. Finally, spend a few moments doing a mock run-through of the activity you're about to engage in. For example, if you're heading out for a run, start with a light jog, or if you're about to play a game of soccer, practice moving sideways, forward, and back. This will give the muscles a "mini-rehearsal," which allows them to practice what they're about to perform, says Fradkin.

125 Go vegetarian for a day

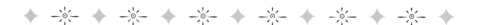

ALL-VEGGIE ALL THE TIME MAY not be your thing, but everyone can benefit from occasionally following a vegetarian diet, says Lalita Kaul, PhD, RD, LDN, and professor at Howard University's College of Medicine. "Vegetarian diets are high in fiber, antioxidants, vitamins, and minerals," says Kaul. Even if you eat vegetables regularly, omitting meat means produce will be the main event at mealtime, not just a side dish.

To make the most of a meat-free meal, don't rely too heavily on starches. Look for dishes made primarily from vegetables or legumes. Leafy green vegetables are a good source of vitamins A, C, and K, and they also contain calcium, folate, and fiber. Remember that the more colorful the foods, the healthier your meal is likely to be, so plan plates with a mix of hues, such as red peppers, yellow corn, green spinach, purple beets, and orange carrots. For protein, tofu is an option, and so are dairy products, like cheese, yogurt, and milk.

126 Try interval training to burn more in less time

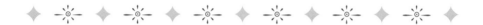

BUSY SCHEDULES OFTEN MEAN you have to squeeze your workout into a lunch hour or a brief break between shuttling the kids around. Optimize this time—and amp up the calories you burn—with interval training. Interval training, in which you alternate pushing yourself with slower, less intense periods, burns more than a steady-paced workout and takes less time. And, according to recent research from Canada's McMaster University, these mini-bursts of speed will also help you to gain strength and endurance faster than a typical workout, as well as make your body more efficient at burning fat. Best of all, while gains have been reported in exercisers who go "all out"—pushing themselves as hard as they can during bike, run, walk, or swim sprints—it turns out that similar results occur when you exercise at a slightly lower intensity, increasing your power output to only an eight, not a ten. To start interval training, use a watch to measure one fifteen-second sprint for every two minutes of less intense exercise. Over time, adjust your rest and sprint periods so that they're closer to the same length.

127 Solve problems without avoidance or ambushes

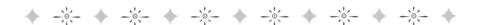

WHEN IT COMES TO CONFLICT resolution, people usually fall into one of two camps: you either want to avoid the conflict in hopes that it will go away, or you jump into it with the intention of solving things as quickly as possible. But neither way is productive for real problem solving, says Lynne Hurdle-Price, president of Hurdle-Price Professionals, a conflict resolution and diversity awareness consulting organization based in the Bronx, New York. The best way to find resolution is by addressing a problem with time and care.

"Conflict resolution is not a fast-food process," says Hurdle-Price. "There is no quick and easy in and out." Start to get perspective on a problem by really listening to the viewpoints of others. Then take time to digest what you've heard. Finally, try to talk through possible solutions. Come up with a few ideas of your own, keeping in mind the various viewpoints of the group, and encourage other people to present their own solutions. According to Hurdle-Price, it takes time, patience, and faith in the process to see results and find better ways to work through problems. But as you learn to work toward solutions that are a better fit for all, you will experience the process with a little less dread.

128 Learn to trust yourself

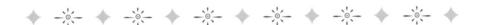

WHEN YOU HAVE TO MAKE A difficult decision, do you call your parents, siblings, and best friend for advice, then follow whatever course of action makes up the majority? While your friends and family have valuable opinions, you already have all of the information and tools necessary to make a good decision; you just need to learn to trust yourself. To become more firm in your convictions, take the time to explore your feelings and gain confidence in yourself, says Parker Palmer, PhD, author of *A Hidden Wholeness: The Journey Toward an Undivided Life* and founder of the Center for Courage and Renewal, an organization devoted to helping people to bring positive change to their lives.

Get perspective on the situation by asking yourself honest and open questions about how you really feel. By recalling past instances in which you've felt the same way and figuring out what your real hopes and fears about a situation are, you'll get closer to the root of your inner emotions. If the thoughts aren't flowing, try journaling to get your ideas out. This sort of inner dialogue will help you access the answers in yourself, says Palmer. Learning to trust what your emotions are telling you is a skill that develops over time, but with practice, you'll be more inclined to ask yourself for the answers, rather than turn to friends for advice.

129 Stand up to slim down

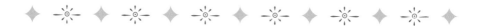

THE MORE YOU SIT, THE MORE likely you are to be overweight. That's the latest from a handful of studies that equate sedentary behavior with not just weight gain, but also an increased risk of several harmful health conditions, including type 2 diabetes and cardiovascular disease. Luckily, separate reports show that just two and a half hours of moderate activity each week can not only help you to drop pounds, but also extend life. Any type of aerobic activity will do, so long as you're exercising at an intense enough level. To tell if you are, take the talking test: you should need to take a breath after every few words you speak when exercising at a

moderate pace. To reap the most benefits, keep your activity high throughout the day, even when you're not explicitly exercising. One of the biggest reasons people don't lose weight after they start working out is that they reduce their everyday activity (such as taking the stairs instead of the elevator) and don't burn as many calories as before. As you start to develop an exercise routine, keep doing your old activities—like taking your dog on long walks, or getting up frequently for water glass refills—to get the best results from your workouts.

130 Addicted to your ex? Just wait it out

ROBERT PALMER WAS ONTO something when he sang, "You know you're gonna have to face it, you're addicted to love." You really can get hooked on the positive side effects of love, like a fast-beating heart and that over-the-moon feeling, but, after getting jilted, you can also suffer from some of the less desirable aspects of addiction, like cravings. Those are the findings of researchers at a trio of New York and New Jersey universities who looked at the brain responses of individuals who'd recently been rejected. When the newly single but still-in-love test subjects looked at photos of their former mates, the part of the brain that responded was the same area that is active when cocaine addicts experience cravings. While there was no immediate way to turn off the response, the strength of the reaction faded throughout the duration of the experiment, indicating that an addiction to a person can be broken, but like any other addiction, it takes time.

131 Learn how to say no

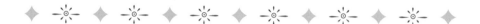

IT'S HAPPENED TO ALL OF US: you get into a conversation with a friend about a charity she's raising money for and before you know it you've not only agreed to attend a silent auction, but you've also been roped into working the event, finding items to donate, and inviting all of your acquaintances. Sure, you'd like to help, but how can you better set boundaries when you're asked to do something you just don't want to do?

"First, recognize that you are a target of persuasion," says Ohio State University psychology professor Richard Petty, PhD. "That will help you mobilize your resources to counter-argue and perhaps recognize the persuasion techniques at work."

In one of Petty's studies, students were asked to agree with an idea they weren't keen on—that they should take an additional exam in order to graduate. Some of the students were told ahead of time that the request would be made; the rest had no forewarning. Not surprisingly, the people who had a bit of advance notice were much better prepared to argue against the idea, while the students who heard the request for the first time were more apt to agree.

Of course, it's not always possible to know when someone is going to try to persuade you, but the next time you're put on the spot, stall for a bit. Rather than answering immediately, insist on a day to consider the request.

132

Set small goals for big results

WHETHER YOU ASPIRE TO RUN a marathon, lose forty-five pounds, or do a full split in yoga class, it's important to have long-term fitness goals. However, keeping these lofty ambitions at the forefront of your mind can be so overwhelming that you actually quit exercising entirely. According to Rodney K. Dishman, PhD, professor of exercise science at the University of Georgia, the best way to ensure your sustained commitment is to aim for smaller, incremental successes in your fitness routine. These will give you direction, and you'll be rewarded frequently with a sense of accomplishment. For example, if your ultimate goal is to be able to bike one hundred miles in a clip, start by setting goals to bike five or ten miles farther than you currently can, and work up to that point. As you meet more goals, your dedication will increase, helping you to set—and reach—larger and larger goals.

133 Get the 411 on food labels

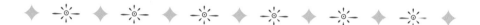

WHAT SHOULD YOU BE LOOKING for when you read the fine print on food labels? People often just skip to the calorie and fat content lines, but that isn't the best way to make choices. "It would be easy to say 'avoid things that provide too much fat, sugar, or sodium,' but if you look at an oil or margarine label, they're 100 percent fat, but can still be part of a healthful diet when used sparingly," says Nancy Cotugna, DrPH, RD, professor of nutrition at the University of Delaware. Fruit juice is another example: juice often has the same amount of sugar,

cup for cup, as a soda, but 100 percent juice also has a good deal of essential nutrients, which makes it a better choice.

Instead of sticking with hard and fast rules, evaluate each food individually in terms of an overall healthful diet, taking into consideration nutrient content, serving size, and, of course, any dietary restrictions. Look at the Daily Value portion of a label, which tabulates the presence of important nutrients such as fiber, iron, calcium, and various vitamins. These summarize the percentage of essential nutrients in an item, and are often a truer measure of a food's worth.

134

Plant your way to peace of mind

GARDENING CAN BOOST THE curbside appeal of your home, but tilling soil and trimming plants can also bring a major dose of stress relief. Take, for example, one study from the Netherlands: thirty test subjects were asked to either garden or read after a stressful situation. Both tasks reduced levels of cortisol, the stress hormone, but the weeders and planters saw greater drops. What's more, when the test subjects were asked how they felt, the gardeners reported feeling fully recovered from the stress, while the people who had read actually reported feeling worse.

So, the next time you need to blow off steam, reach for a trowel. Working the soil, planting seeds or starters, and tending to fully grown plants can help you to bury your stress almost instantly. Also, because both viewing the color green and being in green space have been shown to have positive effects on anxiety, you'll be rewarded by simply being in your garden, as well as by the act of gardening itself.

135 Don't spoil your diet with snacks

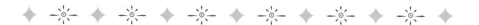

WHEN MIDDAY BOREDOM SETS in, do you reach for a bag of M&M's? According to new research, Americans are snack happy, with 97 percent of the population enjoying in-between-meal treats, a jump from 71 percent in 1977. Snacking isn't a bad thing—many diets tout eating several small meals throughout the day to keep the metabolism working and prevent hunger-fueled binges. But, if you eat several small meals, be sure to keep your total caloric intake at USDA recommendations.

"Snacks add to daily calorie values, which is a problem," says Barry M. Popkin, PhD, professor of nutrition at the University of North Carolina and director of the school's Interdisciplinary Obesity Center. In his studies, he found that, on average, people eat one more snack each day compared to 1977, and snack size has gone up while nutrients have gone down.

Luckily, a few simple changes can help keep your habit—and your health—in check. Avoid packaged snacks advertised as low-calorie, says Popkin, who wrote *The World Is Fat: The Fads, Trends, Policies, and Products That Are Fattening the Human Race.* While these sorts of snacks may be low in calories, they don't offer much to satisfy hunger, leading you to eat more. Instead, look for foods with health benefits, like fruits, vegetables, and whole-grain products with minimal added sugar.

136 Build happiness with each birthday

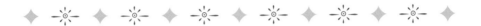

GETTING UP THERE IN YEARS?
Don't worry: According to a new study, self-esteem actually increases over time, building from young adulthood to late middle age. On average, most people feel best about themselves at about sixty years old, says psychology research professor in the University of Basel's department of psychology Ulrich Orth, PhD, co-author of the study, which evaluated people between 25 and 104 years of age.

At four different intervals over sixteen years, the more than three thousand test subjects were asked to rate statements about themselves, such as "I take a positive attitude toward myself," which suggests high self-esteem, and "All in all, I am inclined to feel that I am a failure," which clearly points to low self-esteem. Women had lower levels of self-esteem when they were younger, their scores evened out with men over time, and both saw gains in middle age. Researchers theorize that self-esteem rises after your turbulent twenties and thirties as your life becomes a bit more stable and your status at work and home is elevated.

137 Set aside time for cell phone conversations

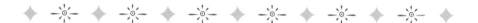

YOU KNOW THAT DRIVING WHILE talking or texting on a cell phone can be distracting and dangerous—that's why there are laws regulating that sort of communication. But new research from the psychology department at Western Washington University shows that talking on a cell phone while *walking* can cause you to miss a lot, too, increasing your risk of getting into an accident as a pedestrian. In the study, a number of people who talked on their cell phones while walking experienced inattentive blindness: during their strolling chat session, they didn't see a unicycling clown that crossed their paths. The implication is that if you're blind to something as outlandish as that spectacle, you're probably also missing a lot of other stuff, too, such as friends you pass, a twenty-dollar bill on the sidewalk, or, perhaps more importantly, traffic signals. Another reason to call when you've got less going on: other studies have shown that being distracted from the call by things around you—like switching your attention from talking to negotiating how to cross a busy street—is usually felt, and at times resented, by the caller on the other end.

138

Choose a deeper massage for deeper benefits

YOU ALREADY KNOW THAT A massage improves your mood and soothes your stress levels, but it turns out that—depending on what type of massage you choose—it can also boost your immune system response. Researchers from Cedars-Sinai's psychiatry and behavioral neurosciences department recently recruited people to experience either forty-five minutes of Swedish massage—a deep type of touch—or forty-five minutes of light-touch massage. Based on blood tests performed right after the gentle and firm styles of rubdown, the people who received a Swedish massage had lower levels of the stress hormone cortisol and an increase in lymphocytes, the white blood cells that help with fighting disease and infection.

139 Stretch to strengthen your heart

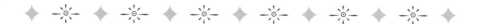

YOU MAY NOT BE ABLE TO DO A split or put your legs behind your head, but there's no need to strive for those fancy feats of flexibility. As it turns out, simply being able to touch your toes is a good indication of your health. According to new research from the University of North Texas, people over forty who passed the sit and reach test—like a seated toe-touch, reaching forward over straight legs—had more flexible arteries than those who couldn't do the stretch. Based on these findings, less-flexible people are more at risk for cardiovascular disease.

A regular stretching routine can increase your range of motion and lower your risk of future heart problems. Aim to stretch a few times each week, being sure to hit your major muscle groups, like your quads, hamstrings, glutes, and chest. Stretches should be static—no bouncing—and are most effective when held for thirty to sixty seconds at a time. Push yourself to the point of discomfort, but not pain.

140 Change your thoughts to make over your mood

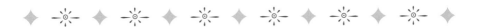

WHEN YOU CAN'T SHAKE NEGA- tive, self-doubting thoughts, you may try to distract yourself by flipping on the TV or going out with friends. This can offer a temporary fix, but to get to the root of the problem, try changing your thoughts before you resort to changing your behavior, says Daniel Strunk, PhD, assistant professor of psychology at Ohio State University. By examining the thoughts that are bringing you down—and looking at them with skepticism and scrutiny—you'll be able to stop the cycle.

"If you have the thought 'No one cares about me,' search for evidence that someone in your life really does care," says Strunk. You'll likely find this evidence, and realize that perhaps the people in your life just aren't showing their care in ways you like or as frequently as you want. As you think through the possibilities, you'll often find that these negative automatic thoughts are actually untrue, or at least a bit inflated, says Strunk. By recognizing these as unrealistic early on, you'll react with a less emotional response and won't get dragged down so deeply.

141

Trade instant gratification for long-term health

IF YOU STRIVE TO LIVE IN THE moment, you're on to something—studies show that being present increases happiness. But if your unwavering focus on the now leads to unhealthy behavior—such as having one more cocktail or skipping a workout—you might need to shift your emphasis away from instant gratification. According to researchers at Kansas State University, people who are able to factor the future into deliberations ultimately make healthier decisions. When the scientists studied the extracurricular behaviors of undergrads, they found that those who weighed the future consequences of a decision—for example, that one extra drink could lead to a hangover or weight gain—were more likely to skip the short-term burst of fun in favor of their long-term health. Spontaneity isn't inherently a bad thing, but if you find it's taking a toll on your health, keep the big picture in mind when you make decisions.

142 Thirty minutes to a better body image

THE NEXT TIME YOU HAVE A "FAT day," head to the gym. You already know that regular exercise helps you tone and trim your body, but according to research conducted by Heather Hausenblas, PhD, associate professor of applied physiology and kinesiology at the University of Florida, just one short workout can give you a better body image.

In a review of fifty-seven studies, Hausenblas found that the simple act of going to the gym or heading out for a walk made people rate their appearances higher than before, even if they didn't experience any measurable changes in their bodies. For best results, try getting thirty minutes of moderate activity five days a week, says Hausenblas, though fitting in any amount—more or less—will help you to feel better about your body.

143 Add flavor to your life with an herb garden

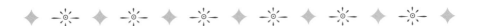

HOME-GROWN HERBS CAN ADD flavor to your meals and cut down on your grocery bill. Even new gardeners can reap the rewards, as many herbs will flourish without a green thumb, according to Mona Laru, ADA, founder of Naked Nutrition, an eating, exercise, and wellness counseling service in the New York area. The plants are compact enough to grow on a windowsill or balcony but potent enough to add a burst of flavor to any meal.

"Parsley, dill, mint, thyme, basil, rosemary, oregano, cilantro, and chives all require minimal space and care," says Laru, "but be sure to check which plants work best in your climate." For best results, purchase seeds in early spring and plant according to the instructions on the back of each packet (if you're behind schedule, simply pick up starter plants in early summer). In addition to best time of year to plant, each seed packet should detail ideal water and sunlight conditions.

After your herb garden has sprouted, experiment with new recipes, suggests Laru. For example, mint can be used in everything from iced tea to a side dish of sugar snap peas or a summer pasta.

144 Take care when choosing a chair

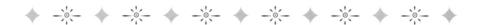

IF IT FEELS LIKE YOU SPEND THE majority of your waking hours seated, you're not alone: the average U.S. adult spends about eight hours of each day sitting, according to the American College of Sports Medicine, and if you work at a desk job, your average may be even higher. Prolonged periods of sitting can lead to serious aches and pains—that's why choosing the right chair is extremely important, says Karen Jacobs, EdD, OTR/L, clinical professor of occupational therapy at Boston University.

When selecting a new desk chair, look for an adjustable model, says Jacobs. A customizable frame will allow you to change the height and depth of the seat as well as the angle of the chair's back. When you fit the chair for your body, make sure your feet

rest squarely on the floor or purchase a foot rest, which is a small riser for the feet. Slide the seat backward or forward so you have about two fingers' width between the front edge of the seat and the back of your knees. Position the chair's back at an angle between 90 and 105 degrees—this will reduce pressure on the spine. When you're seated, be sure to lean back into the chair for support and to give your back muscles a chance to relax.

Of course, the most important way to sit comfortably for long periods of time is to remember to stand up frequently, says Jacobs. She suggests standing up every twenty minutes and taking a few minutes to stretch, refill a water glass, or walk around the office before settling back into your seat for more work.

145

Flowers can draw you out of a funk

NEXT TIME YOU'VE GOT THE blues, think roses. Or violets. Or lilies, daisies, and dahlias, for that matter: simply viewing flowers can instantly boost your mood, according to research performed by Jeannette Haviland-Jones, PhD, professor of psychology at Rutgers University. Flowers and flower scents promote happiness across the board, though receiving flowers seems to be particularly effective. In her studies, Haviland-Jones found that people who were given flowers were more talkative and out-going afterward, reported closer connections, and scored higher on memory tests.

To add a happy focal point to your day, visit a florist or cut some blooms from your garden and place them somewhere you spend a lot of time, like in your kitchen or office. Bet-ter yet, gift flowers to a friend when you're feeling down: you'll pass along the benefits of the blooms while lifting your own spirits with generosity.

146 Tap into the serenity of silence

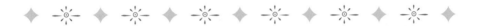

YOU MAY FEEL SOOTHED BY THE silence you find in a forest or at the end of a yoga class. But if you're like most people, silence can seem a little daunting—with no voices or sounds to distract you, you're stuck with your own thoughts. According to Sharon Salzberg, author of *Real Happiness: Learning the Power of Meditation,* most people who sign up for their first silent retreat are more worried than excited. But, she says, they leave with the realization that, "For once in my life, I can be myself. I don't have to be charming or funny—I can just be with my own experience."

You don't have to head off to a full-fledged retreat to benefit from silence. Eating one meal a week without chatter or distraction can help you tap into this calm space, as can setting aside silent time to savor a cup of tea each day. The activity can really be anything you want—the important thing is that you choose to focus your attention solely on what you're doing in that moment, says Salzberg. Without worrying about how others are reacting to you, or diverting yourself with TV or a magazine, you'll be able to focus on the taste of the food, the environment you're in, and any thoughts you have or sensations you feel. This break from everything else will bring you back to yourself.

147 Turn yourself upside down . . . literally

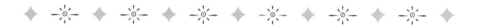

HANDSTANDS MAY SOUND LIKE child's play, but in yoga, going upside down is a regular part of practice. In fact, many instructors believe that inverting your body so that your head is below your heart is one of the ways yoga helps you to keep a young mind and body.

"Physiologically, inversions are believed to reduce blood pressure and assist in bringing fresh blood to the organs and vitality to the whole body," says Julie Dohrman, a certified Anusara yoga teacher in New York City. "On a mental level, inverting is a way to literally get a new perspective on something. It can clear a busy or anxious mind, and allow creative problem solving to resume."

For beginners, Dohrman suggests holding Downward Dog for several breaths. To get into position, move your body into an inverted *V* shape so that your hips point toward the ceiling and your hands and feet are both on the ground, shoulder-width apart with around four feet between toes and palms. More advanced yogis can work on headstands and handstands. To get started, ask a teacher to help you with your technique.

148 Ease your pain through your perceptions

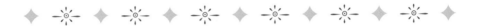

NOBODY *LIKES* GETTING A SHOT from the doctor, but if you're afraid of needles, the prospect may loom large in your mind. And although it's unlikely that you actually have more sensitive skin or a lower pain tolerance than the average person, worrying about pain can cause you to experience it more intensely. According to Chantal Berna, PhD, a researcher in the University of Oxford department of psychiatry, there's strong evidence that anticipatory anxiety and worry about a painful event can increase your level of discomfort.

"Focusing your attention on a painful experience influences your perception of the pain," says Berna. "If someone is paying attention to a painful stimulus, it will feel more intense than if they're distracted by another task, such as a video game." Looking away and humming a favorite tune can reduce feelings of anxiety when going in for a simple medical procedure, like a vaccination. If you have a more complicated visit coming up and you're feeling uneasy, talk to your doctor. Physicians typically have their own strategies for reducing patient fear and worry. Plus, simply understanding the procedure may help you to enter your appointment feeling more relaxed.

149

Get the sun's benefits, not its burn

THE SUN IS OUR GREATEST
source of vitamin D, but sunblock—which
is important for protecting our skin from
ultraviolet rays—actually blocks our ability
to absorb the nutrient, says Hector DeLuca,
PhD, chair of the biochemistry department
at the University of Wisconsin-Madison,
and a leader in vitamin D research. Unfortunately, vitamin D deficiency can cause all
sorts of health problems, from weak bones
to mental decline, cancer, and a number
of autoimmune ailments like heart disease.
To get all the vitamin D you need, take a
supplement, suggests DeLuca. The National
Institutes of Health's recommended daily
allowance falls at around 25 milligrams, but
some studies suggest that a slightly higher
dose is better, so check with your doctor for
a recommendation. You can also up your
intake by eating foods that are fortified with
vitamin D, such as milk or orange juice,
though you'll likely still need a supplement
to meet health recommendations.

150 Think full to feel full

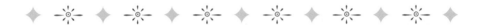

IF YOU'VE EVER FELT HUNGRY after a large meal or full for hours after a light snack, you know your cravings don't always match your consumption. Now, there's an explanation for why: your mind, not your stomach, often determines how full you feel after eating. According to research performed by Jeff Brunstrom, PhD, a behavioral nutrition researcher at the University of Bristol, if you expect to feel satisfied after eating something—anything—you likely will.

In one of Brunstrom's studies, people were shown either a small or a large plate of fruit and then asked to drink a smoothie made from what they'd seen. People who viewed the larger pile of ingredients felt full for longer than those who saw the smaller portion, even though the smoothies were actually made with the same amount of fruit. Likewise, in another study, when people consumed a small bowl of soup—which was secretly being refilled—they felt hungry again soon after, even though they'd already eaten quite a bit.

Our memories about the amount of food we consume influence how hungry we feel after a meal or snack, says Brunstrom. Tricking yourself into eating less is a difficult task, but you can make it easier by slowly shifting your idea of an appropriate portion size. This change in mindset may very well decrease the amount of food it takes for you to feel full.

151

Indulge in art for a happiness boost

NEED AN EXCUSE TO BUY TICKETS for that concert you want to see, or the play that's been getting rave reviews? Here you go: according to Norwegian scientists, the benefits of the arts extend beyond those who are performing, painting, or otherwise tapping into their creativity—even audience members and gallery attendees get the positive effects, which include a boost in mood and higher ratings of self-perceived health. Scientists are unsure what exactly causes these responses, but it may be because involvement in the arts leads to feelings of camaraderie, or because art provides inspiring diversion. If you aren't a singer or sculptor by nature, investigate the types of performances you enjoy and the works of art you appreciate. Simply sitting in the audience or walking through a gallery can help you to feel healthier and happier.

152 Create daily pauses for appreciation

IF MOST OF YOUR INNER DIA-
logue seems to be taken up by to-do lists
and worry, you'd benefit from finding a
way to spend more time thinking about the
things that bring you joy. To do this, says
Linda Lantieri, director of The Inner Resilience Program, an organization focused
on building emotional strength in school
teachers, create rituals around things you
do every day. Choose a few things you do
regularly, like turning on your computer or
brushing your teeth, and attach meaning
to them, using that time to conjure up a
thought or feeling you want more of in
your life.

For example, says Lantieri, each time you put
the key in your front door, take a moment to
be grateful that you have a place of respite to
go each night. When the phone rings, take
the opportunity to stop, take a deep breath,
and thank your body for your health. Or,
each time you pour a cup of coffee, think
about someone in need. By making space
for these moments, your mind shifts from
its usual state of overstimulation into one
that's calm and hopeful. Best of all, these
mini-meditations won't take up any extra
time since the prompts they're attached
to—opening the door, pouring coffee—are
already a part of your day.

153 Forgo fragrance for a toxin-free home

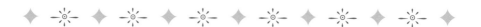

YOU KNOW WHAT A CLEAN home smells like—usually lemon, pine, lavender, or a mix of all three. But these lovely scents could actually be hazardous to your health, says Cassidy Randall, program and outreach coordinator for Women's Voices for the Earth, a watchdog organization for the environment. The ingredients used to make fragrances in many popular household cleaners can cause skin and eye irritations, allergies, and other, more severe conditions.

"In a recent report, we revealed that hidden chemicals in fragrance are potentially linked to hormone imbalance, reduced fertility, and an increased risk of breast cancer," says Randall. Minimize your exposure to these toxins by looking for fragrance-free products, but be aware that products labeled as unscented may actually contain a fragrance to mask the smell of other chemicals. Labels do not always list ingredients (even natural ones, like lavender or lemon oil, which can also be irritants), so research products online, searching for cleaners free of phthalates, synthetic musks, and allergenic fragrance agents.

154 Keep your conversa- tions private

THERE'S A REASON THAT listening to someone yap away on a cell phone hits a nerve: overhearing almost any conversation can be annoying, and listening to just one side of it is actually a lot more distracting than listening to a full discussion, say researchers from Cornell University. Scientists have concluded that when you hear two people talk, the conversation usually flows in a predictable way, which makes it easy for your mind to tune it out. But when you overhear just one end of a conversation, the speaker's words seem more unpredictable, so you may subconsciously strain to hear what's being said, making it harder to focus on something else. Keep this in mind the next time you find yourself irritated by a conversation you find yourself privy to, or the next time you're tempted to pick up your phone in cramped quarters.

155 The healing power of hope

TESTING THE EFFECTIVENESS of healing prayer has proven difficult for the research community: there's just no quantifiable way to measure the strength of a person's positive thoughts, and it's impossible to ensure that people outside of a study aren't skewing the results with prayers of their own. But recent research from Harvard Medical School has demonstrated that simply *believing* someone is praying for you can improve your health. When patients in the study were told they might be prayed for, they all made comparable health gains, regardless of if they were actually being prayed for or not. While this doesn't necessarily confirm the idea that prayer heals, it does reinforce the notion that hope is a powerful tool for overcoming illness. Whatever your circumstances, keep a positive attitude to help your cause.

156

Power nap to boost performance

HOPEFULLY YOU'LL NEVER GET caught napping at work, but if you ever do, just tell your boss that your desk dozing is actually making you smarter! It may sound far-fetched, but that's what researchers from the University of California, Berkeley found in a recent study that tracked how a ninety-minute nap affected people's ability to learn. Before naptime, all of the study participants performed equally well at a task that required learning lots of new information. But after the brain game, only half of them were allowed to nap. When they repeated the drill, those who had slept performed better than those who hadn't, and the nappers scored higher in round two than they had during the first go-around. Scientists say that sleep not only refreshes your brain, but also allows the mind to make more room in your short-term memory banks, which is vital for assimilating new information.

157

Adjust your workout intensity to reach fitness goals

HOW HARD DO YOU PUSH yourself in your workouts? Your answer is more important than you think: different levels of exercise intensity produce different results in your body. If your only exercise goal is to burn calories, then a moderate level of intensity may get you results; but if you're training for a race, or exercising with the intention of gaining more muscle, power, or speed, this is actually the level of intensity you want to avoid. On a scale of one to five, with one being minimal effort and five leaving you breathless, three is what professional mountain bike racer Rebecca Rusch, winner of several world titles, calls "the garbage zone." When you work out at this level, you're exercising too hard to give your body a rest but you aren't pushing yourself enough to make actual gains in strength, says Rusch. Before a workout, decide which it's going to be—a work day or a gentle day—then challenge yourself to stick with it, and not let yourself shift to exercising in the middle.

158

Cut computer time to get creative at work

CHANCES ARE, YOUR JOB requires a lot of computer face-time, whether you're doing research online, corresponding over e-mail, or typing up a report. But if you don't turn your back on technology occasionally, you're likely overloading your frontal cortex, the part of your brain that's responsible for decision making and problem solving, says David Strayer, PhD, professor of psychology at The University of Utah.

To keep from depleting this important resource, Strayer recommends that you take computer, phone, and e-mail breaks. Try to head outside at least once a day, leaving your phone and other gadgets behind: creating that space just may help you find a solution for a problem that's been plaguing you. When it comes to brainstorming, try to have in-person chats as often as you can, rather than e-mail dialogues; you'll be better able to focus on the idea if you don't have one eye on your inbox.

159

Harness group energy to make exercising easier

STUDIES HAVE SHOWN THAT working out with a friend will help you commit to fitness—you're less likely to blow off cycling class if your best friend is there waiting for you—but new research indicates that working out in a group may actually make exercise feel easier, too. According to the research, the bond formed between exercisers in a group causes an increase in pain tolerance, which means you can work out longer and harder. This boost was most pronounced among people who did synchronized sports, such as dancing or rowing, says Emma Cohen, PhD, co-author of the study and an anthropologist at the Max Planck Institute for Evolutionary Anthropology. To walk (or run, or cycle) longer or faster on your next outing, invite a friend: it'll be more fun, and feel like less work.

160 Drink up to boost your mood

IF YOU GET CRANKY IN HOT weather, don't resign yourself to sullen summers—you have more control than you think. Even mild dehydration, which tends to accompany heat, can have a negative effect on mood, say researchers at Boston's Tufts University. During a short bout of sweat-inspiring fitness—enough to cause a 1- to 2-percent loss of fluids, or for most of us 1 to 3 pounds of water weight—some exercisers were given water and others were not. After the workout, the dehydrated exercisers were in a worse mood than the ones who were allowed to drink, and they were also more fatigued and performed less proficiently at memory tests. Of course, dehydration can occur even without exercise, particularly on hot days. To tell if you're drinking enough water, take the toilet test: if your urine is darker than lemonade, you need to consume more fluids.

161 Treat anxiety with activity

SAVE MONEY ON A SHRINK AND join a gym. That's the latest from Michael Otto, PhD, professor of psychology at Boston University and co-author of *Living with Bipolar Disorder: A Guide for Individuals and Families.* "Reports show that exercise is as effective at treating anxiety as interpersonal therapy, cognitive behavioral therapy, and pharmacological therapy, the three main treatments for anxiety." In fact, in a recent report Otto compiled, the evidence was so compelling that he was inspired to jumpstart his own fitness routine. Regular bouts of aerobic activity that bring the heart rate up to around 70 percent of your maximum—such as swimming, jogging, and biking—appear to work best. If that isn't possible, head out for a power walk the next time you feel anxious. Chances are your symptoms may be gone by the time you finish.

162 Hold the salt for better health

REACHING FOR THE SALT SHAKER to flavor a meal may seem like a harmless move, but a few shakes is all it takes to overdo your sodium chloride consumption and increase your risk for high blood pressure and heart disease. According to German researchers, eating or drinking more than 6 grams of salt each day is bad for your health, and most of us get more than twice this amount. Even if you don't add salt to your foods, you're still at risk: most packaged foods—even sweets—are loaded with the ingredient. To cut down on the amount of salt you take in, read nutrition labels to inform your food purchases. Or better yet, prepare more of your own meals. You'll be able to gauge more accurately how much sodium you consume, plus when you use fresh, flavorful ingredients, you'll have less reason to shake on a layer of salt.

163 Cut chemicals from your morning routine

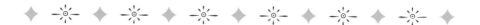

YOU MAY HAVE BECOME MORE savvy about the chemicals you put in your body—think organic veggies and hormone-free meats—but how careful are you about the toxins you put *on* your body? If you aren't reading the labels of your shampoo, lotion, and other toiletries, you're in for a surprise, says Alexandra Spunt, co-author of the book *No More Dirty Looks*, which examines the use of harmful and hazardous chemicals in the beauty industry.

You may remember an uproar a few years ago about paraben, a preservative used in lots of products for the face and body; paraben's use has tapered out, but the chemicals that replaced it aren't much better. "Preservatives like DMDM-hydantoin, imidazolidinyl urea, diazolidinyl urea, and quaternium-15, which are common in skin- and hair-care products, are what are sometimes called 'formaldehyde donors,'"

says Spunt. This means that these ingredients slowly release formaldehyde, which is a carcinogen, into the products and, in turn, onto you. While some toxicologists say that these chemicals only release a small amount of formaldehyde, enough toxin-free products are available today that it's not worth using ones that may be hazardous to your health.

The same goes for products that come with artificial fragrance. These scents may make you smile when you catch a whiff, but because companies don't have to disclose the ingredients that create the smells, there's no telling what goes into them. For example, phthalates, common fragrance chemicals used in face and body care, are hormone disruptors linked to a number of health concerns, says Spunt. Use scent-free products whenever you can.

164 Eat organic on a budget

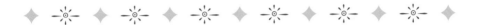

EATING ALL ORGANIC, ALL THE time, gets pricey. Fruits and veggies grown without pesticides are often more expensive than non-organic varieties—sometimes more than double the cost. Luckily, some non-organic fruits and veggies are less dangerous than others. Not all produce is treated with or affected by pesticides in the same way, says Mona Laru, ADA, founder of Naked Nutrition, an eating, exercise, and wellness counseling service in the New York area.

For fruit, it's okay to buy non-organic if a fruit has a thick, inedible skin, such as bananas, avocados, mangos, grapefruits, and pineapples. However, if a fruit has a thin, edible skin, like apples, grapes, berries, and peaches, it's best to buy organic.

Without a thick barrier, more chemicals may be absorbed by the actual fruit. And, because thin-skinned fruits attract more bugs, according to Laru, more chemicals are used.

Bugs tend not to be attracted to more pungent vegetables like broccoli, cauliflower, and asparagus. However, thin-skinned or more delicate vegetables, like bell peppers and spinach, are often coated with chemicals, so for these, it's best to go organic, says Laru. Also buy organic root vegetables and water-rich plants like potatoes, carrots, and celery, which tend to absorb a high degree of chemicals. Buying frozen organic fruits and vegetables, growing your own, or buying from local farms may also help keep costs down, suggests Laru.

165

Vent strategically after an argument

EVERYONE HAS DONE IT—YOU argue with a friend, then reach out to another friend for validation. The more people you get on your side, the more correct you are, right? While a vote of support will help you feel justified in continuing to fight, it probably won't help you solve the problem. Instead, seek the viewpoint of a trusted friend not to win the argument, but to try to see the argument more clearly.

When you reach out for help in a dispute, find a person who you think will be able to shed light on the other person's perspective, says Robert Gould, PhD, chair of the department of conflict resolution at Portland State University. Rather than asking her to take sides, see if she can help you to see where the other person is coming from. Just don't let this information cause you to acquiesce too soon, warns Gould. "Some people give in to other people's perspectives too easily, so use a conversation with a friend to help you discover your own perspective more deeply, too."

166

Strength train for a slim silhouette

KUDOS IF YOU REGULARLY engage in aerobic activity. But to stay strong and slim, you really need to include resistance work, too, says Michele Olson, PhD, professor of exercise science at Auburn University at Montgomery. Extra muscle mass helps keep your metabolism high, gives your body definition, and can actually improve your endurance during cardio sessions. Men will get an obvious boost in muscle mass if they stick with a routine, but women shouldn't worry about bulking up: between high estrogen levels and low levels of testosterone, women tend to tone but not add a lot of extra mass, says Olson.

167

Choose chilled water

LEAVE A PITCHER OF WATER IN the fridge. According to German scientists, drinking cold water raises metabolism enough that ingesting just six cups of the cold stuff could burn up to fifty extra calories a day. That adds up! Another study found that cold water from the tap was less likely to erode plumbing than warm water; this suggests that cool water can have lower levels of lead. Another reason to go for the cold: in research on athletes, scientists have found time and time again that exercisers who drink cool beverages perform longer than those who drink room-temperature refreshments because the liquid naturally cools down the body.

168

Buddy up to boost fitness and self-esteem

FOR A CONFIDENCE BOOST, work out with a buddy. According to new research from Paul Freeman, PhD, a lecturer in the School of Sport and Health Sciences at the University of Exeter, exercising with a friend can help you feel better about your athletic abilities, and you may just perform better, too. In his research, Freeman found that positive interactions found between pairs of exercisers—which range from mild coaching to high fives and whooping—led to gains in enjoyment and actual ability. Of course, not all workout buddies will enhance your experience and improve your game: for best results—whether you're evenly matched in skill or at different levels—keep competition and coaching friendly.

169 Curb colds—and more— with vitamin D

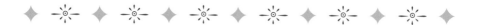

RECENTLY, SCIENTISTS HAVE discovered more and more benefits of vitamin D. This sunlight-derived nutrient is linked to cancer prevention, weight loss, better bone density, and improved brain function, to name a few benefits. It's also a major immunity booster, says Mark Liponis, MD, author of *UltraLongevity*. And yet, a surprising number of people are deficient.

A day in the sun can refill your body's depleted supply and help you stave off colds and more serious conditions, but few people are able to regularly spend enough time outside to maintain proper levels, says Liponis, and sunblock—which is vital— dampens the effects. A supplement is your best option to boost and maintain levels of vitamin D and your immunity. Ask your doctor about the right dosage for you.

170 Regulate your sleep cycle to feel rested

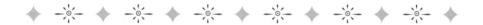

YOU'VE PROBABLY HEARD OF A sleep bank—the idea that you can deposit and withdraw abstract "sleep credits," making deposits on days you have the luxury of sleeping in, and withdrawals when life gets too busy for any real shut-eye. But don't invest too much in this notion: if you zonk out for twelve hours each Sunday in an effort to make up for the five hours a night you get the rest of the week, you're not actually helping your situation.

According to Paul L. Durham, PhD, director of the Center for Biomedical and Life Sciences at Missouri State University, the best way to balance out nights of unrest

is *not* by clocking in more hours of Zs on another night. "When you oversleep, you don't make up for lost sleep," says Durham. "You'll be better off if you try to get the same amount every day."

Seven or eight hours is the recommended amount of sleep for adults, so modify your sleep schedule to make sure you're within an hour or so of this range. And if you're up late one night, don't try to make up for it by sleeping extra the next. According to research, it takes three nights of regular sleep—not one long sleep-binge—to make up for one evening of being sleep-deprived.

171

Love brings on common language

HAVE YOU PICKED UP SOME OF your partner's speech patterns or favorite words? If you're suddenly adopting phrases that are commonly said by your boyfriend, or slipping into your wife's particular intonation of a word, your relationship is likely on solid ground. Psychologists at the University of Texas at Austin recently studied conversations between individuals as well as the poems of famous pairs, including Elizabeth Barrett and Robert Browning. According to their research, a couple starts to use similar language styles and words when they're at their happiest, with similarities and patterns starting to shift when times are troubled. So, as much as you may hate that you now punctuate your questions with an "eh?" or sing certain words more than you speak them, rest assured that picking up the language habits of your other half is actually a good thing.

172

Create healthier cookouts with rosemary

FIRING UP AN OUTDOOR GRILL IS one of the most popular ways to cook meat, but research has found that burgers, steaks, chicken, and other meats cooked over a flame have a large amount of carcinogens—compounds that can contribute to the formation of cancer cells. The good news is that researchers from Kansas State University have found that adding rosemary to your meat or marinades can inhibit the formation of carcinogens by up to 79 percent. If you don't want to alter your perfect rub recipe, simply spread a few drops of rosemary extract on meat before you set it on the grill—the liquid is fairly tasteless, so the flavor will remain unchanged.

173

Squeeze every beauty benefit out of aloe vera

YOU'VE HEARD THAT FRESH ALOE vera can help soothe a sunburn, but that's not the only reason to keep a plant around the house: aloe is an incredible do-everything ingredient that is inexpensive, easy to find, and keeps forever, says Alexandra Spunt, co-author of *No More Dirty Looks*. Aloe vera gel—which oozes out of the plant when it's cut—can also calm rashes, relieve irritation caused by shaving, and even be used as a lotion on the face and body. Plus, just as aloe vera calms the skin, it can also calm down frizzy or dry hair. "Put the aloe juice—which is available in the drinks section of most grocery stores—in a spray bottle and use it on wet hair as a de-frizzer before you blow-dry or air-dry," says Spunt. "As a gel, just a tiny bit of aloe on dry hair will tame and hold without any synthetic plasticizers or silicones." To add shine to hair and tame flyaways the natural way, apply a few drops of natural oil—such as coconut, olive, or jojoba—to dry hair.

174 Drinking diet soda doesn't mean you'll stay thin

IF YOU THINK DRINKING DIET soda doesn't do any harm, guess again. The effects of diet drinks appear to be as bad as—or worse than—their full-calorie counterparts. In a recent study from the University of Texas, zero- or low-calorie carbonated beverages were linked to obesity; the more you drink, the higher your chance of becoming overweight. The connection between weight gain and drinking diet soda isn't entirely clear, but experts suspect that the low-cal version—which can taste even more sugary than regular soda—might make drinkers crave more sweets. And because a beverage isn't as filling as a meal, you may finish a can of cola, then reach for a calorie-laden snack.

175 Eat omegas for increased immunity

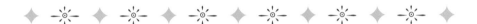

THE MORE OMEGA-3 FATTY ACIDS you consume, the better your immune system works, says Mark Liponis, MD, author of *UltraLongevity*. According to research, a diet high in omega-3 has been linked to lower incidence of heart disease, a healthier mind, and decreased rates of cancer, to name a few benefits. The fatty acids are found in avocados, olives, and other staples of a Mediterranean diet, but one of the easiest ways to up your intake is by adding fish to your menu a couple of times a week.

Omega-3 quantities vary from fish to fish—for example, herring and salmon can have close to 2 grams of the fatty acid in a 3-ounce serving, while mahi mahi and grouper have just .13 grams and .25 grams, respectively. When choosing which fish to eat, it's also important to factor in how susceptible certain types of fish are to environmental contaminants, says Liponis. Small, oily fish generally have lower levels of toxins, such as mercury, than bigger fish. Salmon, sardines, and trout are healthy options. Steer clear of larger fish, like tuna or swordfish.

Fish oil supplements are another way to get your omega-3 fatty acids. Make sure the brand you choose is purified and PCB-free. To find the right dose, talk to your doctor.

176 You are what you do

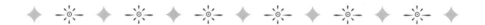

HAVE YOU EVER BEEN SURPRISED to realize that your best intentions aren't shining through in your actions? For example, you may think of yourself as generous because you feel compassion for people less fortunate than you. But if no one sees you acting in a way that reflects those feelings—volunteering at a homeless shelter, or donating money or goods—they may not pick up on your inner dialogue, says Simine Vazire, PhD, assistant professor of psychology at Washington University in St. Louis. The problem, she says, is that we put too much thought on our intentions, but not enough on our actions.

Think about the parts of your personality you'd like others to see, then consider if your actions mirror this. If you can't tell, gauge your friends' reactions to your behavior. For instance, if you think of yourself as reliable, but your friends tease you about being flaky, you may need to rethink how you're acting. "To be seen as the person you think you are, focus on the things you do, not just what you think," says Vazire. "Ask yourself how your actions would come across to someone who doesn't know the 'real' you."

177

Give your workout more weight

ONE OF THE MAIN REASONS people don't get significant results from strength training is because they aren't lifting heavy enough weights. So, if resistance training isn't giving you the firm, defined body you want, it's time to change your routine, says Michele Olson, PhD, professor of exercise science at Auburn University at Montgomery.

"When lifting, the weights should fatigue your muscles in no more than twelve to fifteen repetitions in one set," says Olson. If you can do more reps than that, the amount you're lifting is too light. If those last few reps feel incredibly difficult, try resting longer between sets: recent research has found that taking a three-minute break between sets helped exercisers complete more reps. Keep a log to help you remember which weight is best for each exercise. Remember to date your entries: to get the best results, you should increase the resistance every four to six weeks.

178

Drink herbal teas for your health

NOT ALL TEAS ARE THE SAME.
In fact, the term "tea" can actually describe a number of different beverages. "Black, green, oolong, and white teas are all made by brewing leaves of the plant *Camellia sinensis*, while herbal teas, or tisanes, are made by brewing the parts of other types of plants," says Diane L. McKay, PhD, a scientist at Tufts University's Antioxidants Research Laboratory. Much emphasis has been placed on the disease-inhibiting properties of green and black teas, but herbal teas have considerable health benefits, too. McKay's lab recently demonstrated that drinking three cups of hibiscus tea each day can significantly reduce high blood pressure. And tea that's free of milk and sugar doesn't contain any calories, so replacing calorie-laden beverages—like soda—with tea can actually help promote weight loss, too.

179 Keep your eyes on the prize

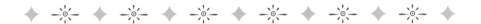

AT THE START OF A YOGA CLASS, an instructor will often ask you to set an intention—to dedicate that day's practice to overcoming a hurdle that's in your path or to a friend in need. But even if you "Om" with your intention in mind, chances are your thoughts will start to wander as soon as you begin moving. Creating a visual reminder will help you to stay focused on your intentions, during yoga class and in life, says Mandy Ingber, a Los Angeles–based yoga instructor.

To put this idea into practice, choose a picture that reminds you of what you want to keep in mind, such as an image of a friend who's battling an illness, or a snapshot that makes you think of the vacation you're taking just as soon as you finish a big project. Put the picture in a visible place—such as at the top of your yoga mat, next to your computer, or inside your medicine cabinet—to remind you to send a prayer, or good energy, or whatever it is you believe in, to that person, idea, or goal. Or, attach meaning to an object you regularly see—such as a tree or your water bottle—so that you start to conjure up the same sort of thoughts each time you see it. Visual reminders like these can help you keep your intention focused in a world full of distractions.

180 Protect your skin like a pro

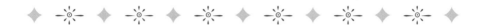

GUARDING YOUR SKIN FROM THE effects of the sun will help fight burns, spots, and wrinkles, but correct sunscreen application is part art, part science, says Sonia Badreshia-Bansal, MD, a dermatologist who teaches at the University of California, San Francisco. Even if you slather on sunscreen every time you step outside, you might not be fully covered. It typically takes about a shotglass full of sunblock to cover your entire body, so be liberal in application, and be sure to spread it right up to the edge of your clothing. Also, reapply at least every two hours while outdoors, says Badreshia-Bansal, and don't forget to protect your lips with an SPF lip balm.

For the best protection, double-check that you're using sunblock, not sunscreen. "Sunblocks are better because they're more broad-spectrum, usable on all skin types, and typically cause less reactions or irritation," says Badreshia-Bansal. Look for a product with zinc oxide or titanium dioxide on its list of ingredients—these offer a high degree of protection and are fairly water resistant—and choose a lotion that's SPF 30 or higher.

181 For health and longevity, go vegetarian the right way

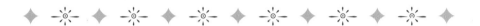

REASONS FOR BECOMING A vegetarian vary greatly—some may give up meat on moral grounds, while others simply may not like how it tastes. From a health standpoint, giving up meat in favor of a more plant-based diet makes sense. In fact, according to Joan Sabaté, MD, DrPH, chair and professor of nutrition at Loma Linda University's School of Public Health, vegetarians have greater longevity and lower risk of heart disease, diabetes, and some cancers.

It's not just about giving up meat, though. A vegetarian needs to make sure to eat a balanced diet to maintain healthy levels of vitamins and nutrients. The Vegetarian Food Guide Pyramid, which Sabaté helped to create, recommends that vegetarians consume fruits and vegetables, whole grains, and beans and legumes at each meal; eat nuts and seeds, plant oils, and egg whites, soy, and dairy daily; and indulge in sweets and eggs only a few times a week.

Sabaté also recommends that vegetarians track their intake of vitamin B12, a brain-boosting nutrient found in animal-derived products, such as meat, eggs, and milk. Too little of this vitamin can cause fatigue, weakness, and even anemia. Lacto-ovo vegetarians may get enough B12 through dairy and egg consumption, and there are several other sources rich in the nutrient including fortified products, such as soy milk and breakfast cereals, or B12 supplements.

182 Break out of a fitness rut

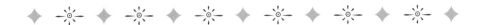

AFTER FOUR TO SIX WEEKS OF the same workout, you may be getting bored—and not just mentally! Your body gets bored, too. The longer you do a particular workout, the more efficient your body gets at it, which means you burn fewer calories and stop making strength gains, according to Phil Cutti, MS, an exercise physiologist in the Human Performance Lab at Stanford University.

Keep challenging your body by varying your routine. If you really like your current workout, try changing the intensity to give your body new challenges. For example, if you strength train, increase the amount of weight you lift or the number of reps, suggests Cutti, or add a few new moves. If you run (or bike, or swim), amp up the pace, change your route, or try interval training.

If you've started to skip workouts, it may be time to try something new. Switch your focus to a different activity, or add a new class or training session to your weekly routine. Taking a break can also cure burnout, says Cutti. Two weeks of rest can rejuvenate your body and mind. When you start exercising again, you'll be challenged by your old workout.

183 Put on rose-colored glasses for better health

IF YOU'RE A GLASS-HALF-FULL person, you already know that life is going to work out okay for you. But if you see the world a bit more pessimistically, a change in attitude may be all you need to start noticing tangible improvements in your life. In one recent study, researchers at four different U.S. universities found that overall optimism slowed the progression of cardiovascular disease and lowered mortality rates while pessimism did the reverse.

Scientists are unsure of whether a positive outlook led to changes in lifestyle, which in turn resulted in improved health, or if attitude itself had an effect on a person's well-being. However, they were able to determine that pessimism leads to greater levels of inflammation, which is one of the causes of cardiovascular disease and other autoimmune diseases.

To protect your health, exercise your ability to look on the bright side. Volunteer, keep a gratitude journal, and limit the amount of time you spend complaining to help you see the world with a bit more hope, and in turn give you even more things to feel good about.

184

Take a multi-pronged approach to sun damage

IF YOU'RE A REGULAR BEACH bum, you know that an umbrella is key for escaping from the blazing sunlight. But while the umbrella's shadow may provide some shelter, it doesn't actually block all of the sun's harmful rays, according to research done at the University of Valencia in Spain.

In a recent study, scientists found that one-third of ultraviolet radiation filters through typical beach umbrellas, which means that even if you're sitting in the shade of one, you're still at risk for sun damage. This doesn't mean you should forgo a beach umbrella—it blocks much of the sun's UV radiation and provides a cool spot to sit—but make sure that you also use standard sun precautions, including sunblock, sunglasses, and sun-shielding hats and clothing.

185

Moderate drinking is best for good health

HERE'S A REASON TO RAISE A glass: Moderate drinking—such as the consumption of one glass of red wine each day if you're a woman, or two beers if you're a man—can have a positive effect on the body, say researchers. In one recent study, scientists at the University of California, Los Angeles found that moderate drinkers were 42 percent less likely die from all causes than heavy drinkers, and 49 percent less likely to die from all causes than alcohol abstainers. Cardiovascular disease and heart attack appear to be two of the main conditions limited alcohol use can protect you from. If you're a non-drinker, it's not too late to get these benefits: in another study, from the University of South Carolina, researchers found that people who went from drinking no alcohol to consuming a moderate amount reduced their risk of developing cardiovascular disease by 38 percent. Taking your drinking habits from heavy to more moderate can also have a positive effect on your health.

186 Respect differences during disagreements

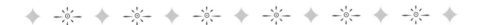

IT CAN BE SURPRISING TO FIND out that a person's opinion on an issue differs from yours, particularly when it's a close friend and a subject you feel strongly about. But if everyone was in agreement all of the time, there'd be no conflict. Reminding yourself that most people you encounter won't share all of your views can help you to keep perspective, which comes in handy when you need to resolve a dispute.

Our views are largely based on a set of deeply personal experiences and identity traits, which include a mix of culture, race, ethnicity, gender, and age, says Lynne Hurdle-Price, president of Hurdle-Price Professionals, a conflict resolution and diversity awareness consulting organization. Because we're all so different, there's a real need for active listening and open questioning when you're trying to reach an agreement. To help better understand where another person is coming from, consider his or her background and what factors may be influencing his or her stance. With all of this in mind, you'll be able to better understand the other person's point of view.

187 Be proactive to beat work burnout

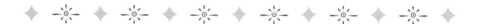

IF YOU'RE FEELING OVERWORKED, your first instinct may be to charge ahead to try and finish faster. But if you don't take the time to regroup, burnout is bound to set in, thwarting your efforts at productivity. Luckily, a few lifestyle changes can help you stay happy while working hard, says Gabriela Corá, MD, MBA, founder of the Executive Health & Wealth Institute in Miami, Florida.

First, get organized, says Corá. To feel like you're accomplishing the items on your agenda, have a list and check off tasks as you do them. Simply seeing that you're making progress can help you stay on track. Time management plays a role, too. Corá suggests planning to do your hardest work in the morning when you're fresh, and scheduling different bits of work into specific times throughout the day.

Once you're able to work more efficiently, you'll have time to fit in mini-breaks, such as lunch. "Eating should be sacred time," says Corá. "So many people are still on the phone or scrolling through e-mails while they eat, but if you can take ten minutes for an interruption-free lunch, you'll gain more energy and be able to work more efficiently." The same goes for exercise—if you start putting in longer hours at the office, don't cut down on your workouts, which can help keep you balanced. While you may be tempted to skip your noon kettlebell class as your workload increases, Corá suggests you do the opposite, adding time to your fitness sessions if possible. Her reasoning: when you're on the brink of burnout, you have an even greater need for the stress-busting benefits of exercise.

188

Nix the iced tea to prevent kidney stones

IF ICED TEA IS YOUR GO-TO thirst-quencher, you may be putting yourself at an increased risk for kidney stones, say researchers at Loyola University Chicago's Stritch School of Medicine. The culprit is oxalate, a chemical found in tea that is key to the formation of the small salt and mineral crystals, which affects about 10 percent of the population. Although hot tea has the same amount of oxalate as iced tea, the chilled form is often consumed in larger quantities; plus, it's popular in warm weather, when you're more likely to be dehydrated, a condition conducive to the formation of kidney stones. If you're an avid iced tea drinker, try to limit yourself to one glass every few days, and be sure to drink plenty of water to help flush away the salt and mineral deposits. Also, sip some fresh lemonade or water with lemon wedges: research has shown that the citrates in lemons actually inhibit the growth of kidney stones.

189 Stay active to alleviate arthritis pain

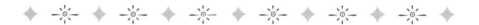

IT SEEMS COUNTERINTUITIVE, BUT if you suffer from creaky, stiff, and painful joints, you may need to exercise *more*, not less. "The only thing that's really been proven to prevent arthritis from acting up is staying active and keeping your weight down," says Gregory S. DiFelice, an orthopedic surgeon at New York City's Hospital for Special Surgery.

Regular exercise can help relieve pressure on the joints by strengthening the surrounding muscles and by contributing to weight loss. Stretching and physical activity also ensure that the joints stay mobile and can help ward off that "stiff" feeling experienced by arthritis sufferers.

Don't be afraid to try new forms of exercise, particularly if the sports you did when you were younger now put the body through a lot of wear and tear. In lieu of high-impact activities like running, try joint-friendly exercise like swimming, which is much better tolerated by arthritis sufferers because of the buoyancy of the water.

190 The right kind of practice makes perfect

IF YOU WANT TO IMPROVE YOUR athletic performance at a specific move, such as your backhand shot in tennis or your Warrior III pose in yoga, it may seem logical to repeat that one action on its own. But new research shows that such focused training actually provides worse results than running through more varied drills, like alternating forehand and backhand shots during a lively tennis volley. According to researchers at the University of Southern California and the University of California, Los Angeles, if you repeat the same motion again and again, you actually don't absorb it deeply. But, if you integrate it into a more complex routine, similar to the sequence of motions you'd usually find it in—such as flowing from one yoga pose to another and another—you'll be more likely to improve the specific move.

191 Write for reflection

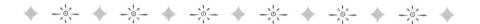

LIFE THROWS A LOT OF CURVE-
balls our way. When you need help making a
decision, clarifying a path, or grappling with
some of life's big questions, it helps to write
down your thoughts. "Writing and thinking
go hand in hand and when we write what's
on our mind, our mind becomes clearer,"
says James Kullander, program curriculum
developer at the Omega Institute for Holistic
Studies, a mind-body focused retreat center
located in New York, and a writer who has
taught workshops on writing as meditation.
"When our thoughts become clearer, so does
our communication."

According to Kullander, writing can help
you to better see who you are, and who you
are not. "When you write from the heart,
your words become richer, more true, and
more transparent," says Kullander.

To make writing come more naturally,
practice even when you aren't trying to sort
through an issue. Kullander suggests you
either focus on the world around you when
you sit down to write, or pay attention to
how you're feeling. If you're stuck, simply
write a description of something, such
as the noise in your kitchen or what you
looked like when you first woke up. "Writing like this helps train the mind to pay
attention," says Kullander. The more you
notice, the more tuned in you'll be to what
you're feeling and thinking, too.

192 Measure your fitness gains

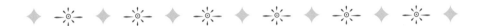

WHETHER YOU'RE IN SHAPE OR about to start an exercise regimen, a little friendly competition can inspire you to give each workout your all, says Pete Cerqua, a personal trainer in New York and author of *The 90-Second Fitness Solution*. Your opponent: yourself. Take five minutes to measure and record the results of the following quick drills. After a month, remeasure to see where you've improved. If your data stays the same, consider increasing the challenge or frequency of your workouts.

FITNESS SELF-TEST

1. Record the amount of time that you can hold a plank and a wall squat. As you get more fit, these numbers should go up.
2. Measure your base heart rate, then measure the change after walking briskly for a minute. Once you're stronger, challenges like this won't cause a significant spike in heart rate.
3. Notice if your knees ache while walking down a set of stairs. Studies show that exercise is one of the most effective ways to end joint pain. After a month of working out, any pain you experience should lessen.

193

Help others to boost your happiness

TURNS OUT YOU GET MORE than a tax write-off when you donate money to charity—you also get a major boost in happiness, according to researchers at The University of British Columbia. A recent study on spending habits found that the more money people spent on others, instead of on themselves, the better they felt. There are limitless ways to be generous, from writing a check to a local women's shelter to taking a friend out for dinner. Of course, non-financial acts of kindness can also help lift your blues, so don't let a shortage of cash keep you from acting with abundance.

194

Get energized in the great outdoors

IF YOU'VE EVER FELT REJUVE-nated after a day spent outside, there's good reason: in a recent study co-authored by Richard M. Ryan, PhD and professor of psychology, psychiatry, and education at the University of Rochester, people who simply spent time in nature experienced a boost in mood and energy. Take a nature break the next time you start to feel slug-gish or stressed. On pleasant days, move an indoor activity outside. For example read your favorite book in the park, not on your couch. When the weather turns, it's still important to get outside. So, bundle up and soak up the nature around you as you walk to the mailbox or shovel snow.

195 Hit the gym for a lifetime of great sex

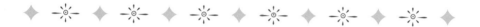

HERE'S ANOTHER REASON TO maintain your health: you'll enjoy sex longer. According to research out of the University of Chicago, men's sexual activity starts to taper off at around age seventy, and women begin to slow down after age sixty-six. But men and women who were healthier than average enjoyed sex for six or seven years longer than those who had more medical concerns, and they were also more interested in sex.

This study cited physical fitness as a main marker for health, and a pile of other research has also shown that exercise can increase sexual satisfaction, interest, and ability for people of all ages. Although there are workouts specifically designed to improve your sex life—yoga for sex, anyone?—following a regular exercise routine of any sort appears to bump up interest in sex, and other studies have shown that working out can lead to more frequent trysts and increased sexual stamina, too.

The next time you want to skip a session at the gym, just think about the benefits fitness can bring to your sex life, now and in the future.

196

Beat belly fat with exercise

HAVE YOU EVER JUSTIFIED excess pounds by explaining that you're naturally "big-boned," or that carrying a little extra weight runs in your family? Sorry to take away your convenient excuse, but new research shows that when it comes to body fat, activity overrides genetics. A Finnish study focusing on twins found that the siblings who were more active had 50 percent less belly fat than their sedentary twins, proving that lifestyle is a bigger predictor of a wide waist than heredity. Over the thirty-seven-year study, the thinner twins fit in an average of one hour of moderate activity each day—such as circuit training, cycling, or walking—while their less fit siblings generally did next to none. That means that sixty minutes of exercise a day will not only help you achieve that sexy flat belly you want, but also cut your risk of type 2 diabetes, heart disease, and dementia dramatically, since all are associated with a rounder middle.

197 Soak away your stress

IF A LONG, STRESSFUL DAY HAS you filling up the tub for a tension-reducing soak, your instincts are right on: according to one recent study from France, bathing as therapy actually outperformed the relaxing effects of a prescription anti-anxiety drug. While the research was conducted at an actual spa, there's no reason you can't replicate the results at home. Simply set aside twenty to sixty minutes of tub time to help your body and mind unwind. To increase your relaxation, add a few drops of a calming essential oil, like lavender, to your bath water, and turn on favorite tunes—inhaling a soothing scent and listening to music you like have also been proven to lift your mood and erase anxiety.

198 Use exercise as a chill pill

DOES YOUR DAILY COMMUTE make you steaming mad? Exercise may be just the thing you need to combat road rage, nagging in-laws, or anything else that makes your blood boil. Recent research found that thirty minutes of cycling at a moderate intensity helped dull anger responses. To keep your cool during trying situations, hit the gym or regularly run around the block—any type of exercise that leaves you a little breathless will provide anger-cooling effects in the moment and over time.

199 Get fresher-smelling feet

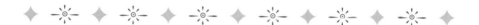

IF YOU'VE NOTICED THAT A PAIR of your shoes is starting to smell, chances are that that not-so-sweet scent will soon spread to your other shoes. This odor is caused by a type of bacteria that thrives in dark, moist spaces—like on feet and in shoes—and can easily be passed from pair to pair. Embarrassing, yes, but this pesky problem is quite treatable. For a chemical-free solution, turn to essential oils.

Tea tree and lemongrass essential oils are antiviral, antibacterial, and antifungal, which means they kill the odor-causing bacteria fast, says Hope Gillerman, a holistic healer and creator of a line of essential oil–based remedies and care products. To eradicate odor in shoes, Gillerman suggests putting a couple of drops of the essential oil inside each pair—a small spritzer bottle can help distribute the liquid evenly. To kill bacteria breeding on the feet, wipe the toes and feet with a damp washcloth infused with a few drops of the oil, or add half of a teaspoon of the essential oil to a small bottle of castile soap to create a bacteria-killing foot wash. Treat shoes and feet every day until the odor disappears. Once the bacteria have been wiped out, you can use the essential oils less frequently.

200 Breathe your way to better posture

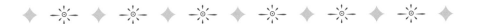

SORE SHOULDERS AND NECK?
You're not alone: a recent survey found that a majority of office workers share this discomfort. A lot of us tighten our necks and shoulders due to poor posture, repetitive movement patterns, or plain old stress, says Joan Arnold, a certified teacher of the Alexander Technique in New York City. Luckily, a little body awareness can help.

To find a release, try this daily breathing practice, suggests Arnold: Lie on your back with a small pillow under your head, your knees bent, and your feet flat. Take a deep breath, letting the inhale be effortless and using the exhale to fully purge the body of air. Imagine that you are filling the back of your body with breath, pressing the back of your ribcage into the floor. As you breathe, reach one hand up to feel your neck—if it's tense, try to relax it. Continue for a few minutes, then practice the same type of breathing the rest of the day: whether standing or sitting, take deep breaths into the back of the ribcage and check the tension in the neck to ease upper body aches.

201 Broach difficult subjects through art

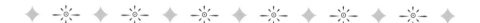

SOME CONVERSATIONS ARE HARD to start, particularly ones that involve painful experiences or deep emotions. To find a way to discuss tough topics or encourage those close to you open up, you needn't share exact experiences, says Parker Palmer, PhD, author of *A Hidden Wholeness: The Journey Toward an Undivided Life* and founder of the Center for Courage and Renewal, an organization devoted to helping people to bring positive change to their lives. "By exploring great questions through poetry and art, you'll be able to create a safe space in which you can share and learn," says Palmer.

"In my work, if another person and I have agreed to discuss something very painful like failure or low self-esteem or abuse, where it's hard to create safe space for talk, I might find a powerful poem that carries that subject, put it between us, and say 'let's explore,'" says Palmer. You may start by talking about a line of poetry that speaks to you in a particular way, or sharing how a painting or sculpture makes you feel. These "third things"—external objects that you can be in dialogue with and about—allow you to say a great deal about yourself without necessarily bringing up specific feelings or experiences you've had, says Palmer. This kind of gentle exploration will allow you to talk about a great range of things, including ideas and topics you never thought you could discuss.

202 Season foods with health-enhancing herbs

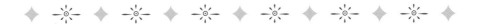

FLAVORING YOUR FOODS WITH salt can put you at risk for high blood pressure, but, there's an easy way to enhance the taste of your meals without adding sodium, fat, or even many calories. "Fresh and dried herbs are packed with flavor, which means a little goes a long way," says Mona Laru, ADA, founder of Naked Nutrition, an eating, exercise, and wellness counseling service in the New York area. A few sprinkles may add just the kick you're looking for.

But the benefits don't end with taste: herbs are packed with antioxidants, which means these plants may help protect against heart disease and cancer, and some—like turmeric and ginger—have anti-inflammatory properties. You can use herbs fresh or dried, says Laru, and you can grow many at home, so you always have a handful available.

To maximize both taste and health benefits, Laru suggests using garlic, cinnamon, and turmeric. Garlic contains anticancer properties and can also reduce risk of cardiovascular disease, says Laru. If you aren't in the mood to cook, add a diced clove to a salad or spread a couple of roasted cloves on a sandwich. Cinnamon, which helps control blood sugar, inflammation, and cholesterol, can be sprinkled on fruit, added to coffee, or mixed into oatmeal. For turmeric, ½ teaspoon a day will spice up fish or a curry dish, in addition to building the immune system and enhancing cancer protection.

203 Add meaning to mealtime with a first course of gratitude

IF YOU'RE NOT RELIGIOUS, YOU may not regularly bless each meal you eat. But, according to Ayurvedic medicine teacher and co-founder of the Deep Yoga School of Healing Arts in San Diego Laura Plumb, "Nature gives us exactly what we need, and that alone is reason to be grateful for your food." This doesn't need to be as ceremonial as saying a traditional grace: simply pause for a moment before you eat to give thanks for the nourishment. "This is a time to remember that food is what we are made of," says Plumb. "Your next breakfast, lunch, or dinner will fuel your body and actually become a part of you, so choose wisely and give thanks."

204 The best (and worst) conversation starters

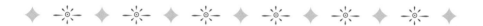

IF YOUR CONVERSATIONS TEND to revolve around items you just purchased, like your new flat screen TV or designer duds, you may not be the life of the party: materialistic people tend to be less popular than those who spend their money on experiences, according to a new study.

Research has long shown that people who value material items over all else usually have fewer and less-satisfying relationships. But one of the latest studies on this topic, co-authored by Thomas Gilovich, PhD, professor and chair of the psychology department at Cornell University, found that people showed aversion to materialistic folk within the first fifteen minutes of meeting them.

In the experiment, subjects started conversations with strangers and talked about either an experience or a possession. The people who talked about their experiences—like a trip they'd recently taken, or a book they enjoyed reading—were more likable than those who talked about their recent purchases. Part of this comes from the type of conversation experiences inspire—that sort of dialogue is typically less about one-upmanship than talk of what a person has bought. "When people talk about their experiences, they enjoy it and enjoy the conversation more than they do when talking about material things," says Gilovich. This enhances the experience for everyone, and causes the listener to like the speaker more.

205 Get fit on the job

STUDIES SHOW THAT OFFICE-based exercise programs improve the health and productivity of workers, but what are your options if your job doesn't have an on-site gym? Plenty, says Rodney K. Dishman, PhD, professor of exercise science at the University of Georgia. Since you probably won't be able to convince your employer to shell out the money needed to build a full-scale workout center, Dishman suggests researching low-overhead programs, like hiring an instructor to come in and teach yoga or Pilates a few times a week. If your bosses don't want to pay, consider splitting costs with other interested colleagues— by bringing fitness straight to you, you're more likely to work out. Or, join or form a company-sponsored sports team, such as a softball league. According to Dishman, group activities like these provide the social support that's vital for starting and sustaining a new fitness program.

206 Dine alfresco for mealtime satisfaction

YOU'VE HEARD OF THE BENEFITS of mindful eating, but paying attention to your food is often easier said than done. Luckily, there's a quick fix: if you have a hard time focusing on your food while you eat, move your meal outdoors, says Sarah Livia Szekely Brightwood, who runs Rancho La Puerta, a popular retreat in Mexico with a renowned garden and cooking school. When you eat outdoors, your senses are nourished by the sights, sounds, and smells of nature, says Brightwood. As a result, you're fully awake and engaged in the moment, which helps you to slow down, savor the meal, and ultimately eat less to feel satisfied.

207 Affirm your appreciation with written thanks

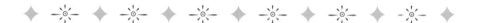

BE HONEST: WHEN'S THE LAST time you sent someone a thank-you note? If the recipient in question was your great-aunt Edie, and the card was mailed after your sweet sixteen party, it's time to break out the stationery. "You can't go wrong sending a thank-you note," says Vicky Oliver, an etiquette expert and author of *301 Smart Answers to Tough Interview Questions*. In this day and age, people have stopped expecting a written acknowledgment of appreciation for occasions big and small, which makes it all the more meaningful to receive one.

"Thank-you e-mails fade seconds after they're opened, but a written note shows that you took extra time and care in your communication," says Oliver. So, when expressing gratitude for a gift that you've been given, put a pen to paper.

Still, this old-fashioned form of thanks is only appropriate in certain situations: for social occasions, go ahead and warm someone's heart with a written note, but opt for an e-mail thanks—which will be delivered more quickly—in business settings. "If you're thanking someone for interviewing you for a job, write an e-mail in the same formal language as a handwritten note," says Oliver. "And, be sure to use spell-check before you hit 'send.'"

208 Stick with your workout

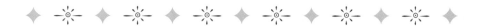

YOU START AN EXERCISE PLAN with a ton of enthusiasm, but five days into it, you skip a workout to socialize; and three days later, you're tired so you watch TV instead. Soon, your fitness routine is 80 percent good intention, but only 20 percent actual working out. What gives? You may not have set yourself up for success, says Ryan Rhodes, PhD, director of the Behavioral Medicine Lab at Canada's University of Victoria. Luckily, a few changes are all it takes to stick with a plan.

First and foremost, find an activity you enjoy. "Chances are that if you're tired, exercise is the first thing you're going to blow off if you don't really like the type of fitness you're doing," says Rhodes. Try to make exercise more pleasurable. Jog on a treadmill in front of the TV, listen to music or a book on tape, or chat with a friend while you walk.

It also helps to remove any barriers to fitness. If you frantically rush out the door in the morning, pack your gym bag the night before; or, if you find yourself drifting toward the couch during your allotted exercise time, hide the remote so flipping channels isn't quite so automatic. Finally, put exercise on your calendar several days each week. Finding the time may be hard at first, but after a few weeks of making space, it will become routine, making it easier to stick with exercise.

209 Speed up your decision time with video games

VIDEO GAMES MAY HAVE STARTED out as a distraction for kids, but more and more adults are getting in on the action. And, it's not just guys—according to one recent study, up to 50 percent of women in the United States play games, too, thanks to the convenience of play on computers and smartphones, in addition to living room–based systems. But is all this virtual sport a waste of time? Not necessarily, say researchers from the University of Rochester. The cognitive scientists found that video game play heightened people's sensitivity to what was going on around them. In fact, after fifty hours of play (broken up over many days), people were able to answer questions and make decisions up to 25 percent faster. And, they were as likely to be right as before the game play, when they were moving a little slower. Scientists think that this result came because video game players are more used to making split-second decisions.

210 Dance your way into her heart

SCIENCE HAS FINALLY PROVEN what anyone who's been to a dance club has long known: ladies like men with moves. A group of researchers in the United Kingdom asked women to rate the dancing styles of nineteen men. The men who had the flashiest steps and incorporated movements for the head, neck, and torso into the dance scored the highest ratings, while the men who incorporated smaller gestures into their steps didn't rate as well. Researchers liken dancing to a mating ritual: as in nature, the showiest males often make the best impression. So fellas, get practicing. And ladies, it's okay to fall for a guy's fancy footwork, just make sure his off-the-dance-floor moves measure up, too.

211

Organize your eating order to stay slim

IF SOMEONE SETS DOWN A FULL plate of pasta in front of you, you may be tempted to push aside your half-eaten salad and dig in. But finishing your veggies first will provide your body with more nutrients, according to research from the University of Florida. In a study that tracked the eating habits of average-weight and obese people, both groups ate the same number of calories, but the difference in intake became clear when researchers tallied exactly what had been eaten: those in the overweight group had consumed fewer plant-based foods and more saturated fats, while those in the average-weight group took in calories that were better for their bodies: namely veggies, fruits, legumes, and whole grains, which supply nutrients and naturally reduce inflammation. Focus on finishing your meals in order of healthiest to least-healthy foods—that way, if you're satisfied before you've cleaned your plate, it will be on the best foods for your body.

212 Stay busy to stay happy, but plan in breaks

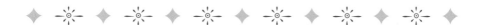

YOU MAY FEEL HARRIED AFTER A jam-packed day—shuttling the kids around, attending appointments, and running errands—but you're likely to be happier than you would be without all of those activities. Those are the latest findings from the University of Chicago, where researchers measured mood in relation to how occupied a person stays. In the study, people were given free time between set tasks, or asked to stay busy for the duration. When the moods of both groups were rated, the people who were occupied the whole time felt better than the ones who had time to kill. Scientists think that this reaction came about because the busier group felt more productive, even though some of the tasks were trivial. While this explains why many of us fill our calendars to the brim, it's not necessarily a positive trait. Being over-scheduled builds up anxiety and stress, so be sure to plan breaks into your schedule, too—listen to your favorite song, go for a stroll, or treat yourself to ten minutes of sitting in the coffee shop after you buy your morning latte.

213

What doesn't kill you does indeed make you stronger

FILE THIS UNDER COUNTER-intuitive but true: if back pain is just one of many hardships you face, you're actually in luck. Researchers at the University of California, Irvine, and the University of Buffalo recently found that having adversity in your life can minimize chronic back pain. In the study, 366 chronic back pain sufferers were surveyed on physical impairment, number of doctor visits, and adverse life events, such as general stresses, relationship problems, or experiencing the death of a loved one. The people who had dealt with more obstacles and misfortune used fewer pain medications, saw their doctors less frequently, and were less likely to report that back pain got in the way of day-to-day life. Scientists believe that adverse conditions may actually toughen you up over time, making you better prepared to deal with less-than-ideal situations, like back pain, when they arise. So if you're feeling low right now, take heart—the experience will only make you better able to handle whatever life throws at you next.

214 Boost your fitness with breath

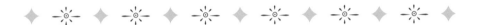

IT'S A FEW MINUTES INTO YOUR workout and you're already out of breath—while your body is ready to keep running, your lungs are panting "slow down" or, more exactly, "stop!" What gives? Your respiratory strength—or your ability to breathe easily under stressful conditions—may not match your physical strength.

Strengthening your respiratory muscles will allow you to work out longer and harder without getting winded. "Most respiratory muscle activity is automatic, involuntary, and continuous," says Thomas Vanhecke, MD, a cardiologist at William Beaumont Hospital in Royal Oak, Michigan, "but controlled breathing can override this." Activities that emphasize control of breath,

including Pilates, yoga, and Tai Chi, can increase respiratory fitness and also improve posture, which is integral to optimal respiratory fitness, says Vanhecke. What's more, when you breathe more efficiently, you spend less energy on your inhales and leave more energy for movement.

To train your breath, you can also focus on your breathing while swimming laps or jogging, trying to breathe at a rhythmic pace. Vanhecke suggests working at the intensity at which talking becomes difficult. Over time, this practice will increase your respiratory fitness, allowing you to work out at a greater intensity without losing your breath.

215 Grow your appreciation for food with a garden

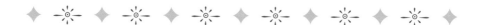

IF YOU STRUGGLE WITH FOOD issues, you may find solace in growing your own. A garden can help you to change how you think about food, simply by reminding you of what food actually is—a source of sustenance that comes out of the earth, says Sarah Livia Szekely Brightwood, who runs Rancho La Puerta, a popular retreat in Mexico with a renowned garden and cooking school. If the majority of the food you eat is processed and packaged, you may think of food in terms of pizza and mac and cheese rather than tomatoes, apples, or lettuce. By planting, harvesting, and preparing your own fruits and vegetables into snacks and meals, you'll rethink your relationship with food. You may find that the foods you make have more flavor, that you appreciate individual ingredients more, or that the act of gardening or cooking lifts your mood enough that you're less tempted to reach for a second helping. According to Brightwood, composting can also help increase your connection with what you eat. As with life, when you realize that you can get rid of the parts you don't want, put them back in the ground, and create something fresh, it's easier to let go.

216 Stop migraines with more sleep

IF YOU SUFFER FROM MIGRAINE headaches, you've probably tried every alleged remedy out there, from medication to meditation. But, according to Paul L. Durham, PhD, director of the Center for Biomedical and Life Sciences at Missouri State University, simply getting enough sleep may be the best means of prevention.

Our bodies produce inflammatory molecules when it's time to rise and shine, says Durham. That's why you may find you get warmer when it's near waking time—your body is literally heating up its engines for a new day. For migraine sufferers, sleep deprivation can cause these inflammatory molecules to over-respond, prompting a migraine attack. Get enough sleep and your body's responses will even out, giving your head more of a chance to stay pain-free.

217 Get svelte on the cheap with a pedometer

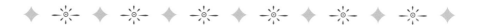

A HEALTH CLUB MEMBERSHIP CAN be expensive, and building a home gym can add up. But invest in a pedometer—a step tracker that can go for as low as ten dollars—and your physical fitness will increase while your weight and blood pressure go down. Those were the results in a recent study from Arizona State University: researchers found that simply wearing a pedometer brought health gains, likely because being aware of your activity levels allows you to set measurable goals around increasing your step count and keeping it high. In a separate study from the United Kingdom, researchers found that people who wore pedometers were able to lower glucose levels—or the amount of sugar in the blood—by 15 percent, enough to reduce risk of type 2 diabetes.

Once you've set up your pedometer, take it for a test spin: wear it for a full week, recording your step count at the end of each day. The next week, aim to up your daily step count by five hundred paces. Continue increasing your steps until you hit ten thousand, the recommended daily step count for health maintenance and weight loss, which is equal to about five miles. To stay motivated, challenge yourself to hit a certain number or start friendly competitions with your friends and family.

218

Put an end to waffling over decisions

IF YOU'RE SECOND-GUESSING yourself about a choice you just made, head for the sink for a quick regret-rinse-off. Recent research from psychologists at the University of Michigan found that the simple act of washing your hands can help you to stop questioning your judgment. While the decisions being made in the study were trivial—ranking preference of one CD over another—this act of "cleaning the slate" by washing your hands may work to help you gain confidence in the bigger choices you encounter, too, like deciding which car to buy, or when to have a difficult conversation.

219 Sweat yourself happy

IF YOU NEED A QUICK PICK-ME-UP, simply slip on your running shoes. Just twenty minutes of aerobic activity can boost your mood, according to a recent study from The University of Vermont, and this positive mindset can last for up to twenty-four hours. Exercisers rode a stationary bike at a moderate intensity for twenty minutes, then rated their levels of various emotions, including tension, anger, and depression, several times throughout the day. For more than a full day after the mini-workout, the cyclists' ratings indicated that they had higher levels of positive emotions and lower levels of negative emotions than the non-exercisers.

In addition to taking your mind off worries and boosting your health, exercise releases mood-boosting endorphins in your brain, which leads to increased feelings of happiness.

220 Get clean sans chemicals

AFTER A WORKOUT OR A LONG day of travel, nothing beats that squeaky clean feeling you get from lathering up in the shower. But, even if the shampoos and soaps you use make your skin and hair feel soft, they may contain chemicals that are hazardous to your health, says Siobhan O'Connor, co-author of the book *No More Dirty Looks*, which examines the lack of regulation in the beauty industry. "Avoid shampoos and body washes that contain sulfates," says O'Connor. "These chemicals are so harsh on skin that they strip beneficial oils and can cause reactions in a lot of people. They can also be contaminated with a chemical called 1,4-dioxane, which is a carcinogen." Once you find sulfate-free cleansers, there's no reason to scrub everywhere, every day: according to O'Connor, your body naturally balances itself with oils, so concentrate on cleaning your essential areas regularly, but the rest of your body should be fine with a quick rinse.

221 Play for better health

IMPROVING YOUR HEALTH CAN feel like work, particularly when it involves adding activities you don't enjoy to your schedule, such as annual exams with your physician. But researchers at Canisius College have found one health-boosting habit that should be easy to stick with: playing more. Reserving time for activities you enjoy doing will help your brain recharge and it can also have positive effects on your body: as your anxiety decreases, elevated blood pressure will even out, too. Play comes in many forms. Some people like to join in a friendly water balloon fight, while others would prefer to cheer on the players. Whatever it is, you'll know when you find it. When you're engaged in play, it will start to feel like your other worries are fading away.

222 Lower your cholesterol the natural way

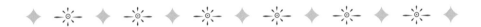

ACCORDING TO THE U.S. DEPART-ment of Health and Human Services, more than sixty-five million Americans suffer from high blood pressure. This condition causes hardening of the arteries and raises the risk of heart disease significantly. Medications can help to control high blood pressure, but, suggests Ronald L. Hoffman, MD, a practicing physician and author of *How to Talk With Your Doctor*, rather than play "cholesterol limbo" with drugs, a better option is to focus on a healthy diet and exercise.

Foods high in cholesterol and saturated fat—like butter and some salad dressings and desserts—can raise cholesterol levels, so limit your daily intake and substitute mono-unsaturated fats, like those found in olive oil. Fibrous foods like vegetables, fruits, and legumes naturally lower LDL cholesterol levels (also known as bad cholesterol), and so do lean proteins, such as fish or soy.

Weight loss will also help lower levels of bad cholesterol and raise levels of HDL, or good cholesterol, says Hoffman. Regular exercise for thirty minutes a day can offer the same rewards. If you're at risk of high cholesterol or already suffering from the condition, make an appointment with your physician to discuss non-pharmaceutical options to get your health back on track.

223 Unplug to beat technology addiction

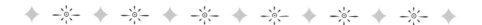

YOU LOVE BEING ABLE TO contact friends and family, check the bus schedule, or look up an address with just the click of a button—but our hyper-connected world has its downsides, too. Technology is a double-edged sword, says David Strayer, PhD, professor of psychology at The University of Utah. Modern breakthroughs enable us to do things we couldn't otherwise, but at the same time, many technologies have the capability of creating addictive behaviors.

Not convinced that you're a technology junkie? Just think about how quickly you reach for your phone when a call or text comes through, or how frequently you check for new e-mails on your computer, even when your workday is done. According to research, those behaviors activate the same region of the brain that gambling addiction stimulates, indicating that you actually become dependent on technology, says Strayer.

To shed this invisible burden, scrutinize your technology use and adjust it accordingly. For instance, if your e-mail sounds an alert each time you get a new message, turn that function off and instead, set a few specific times to check e-mail each day, so you lessen your technological ties a bit. Or, if you must take your cell phone with you when you go for a walk, set it on silent mode, so you can call out if you need to, but you won't be distracted by incoming calls. And be sure to create opportunities to unwind every so often, whether it's a long weekend in the woods (and out of cell phone service areas), or just setting specific hours of the day you keep your computer turned off.

224 Snack smarter

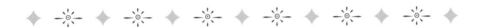

A COUPLE OF HANDFULS OF walnuts seems like an appropriate snack choice: walnuts are full of amino acids and omega-3 essential fatty acids, the good fat that decreases the risk of cardiovascular disease and improves brain function. But, a recent study from Greece found that people who ate a high-fat snack—in this case 100 grams of walnuts—felt hungry faster than those who loaded up on the same number of calories of carbs or protein.

If you're looking for a snack that will tide you over for hours, "opt for foods rich in protein and complex carbohydrates," says Alexander Kokkinos, MD, PhD, lecturer of internal medicine at the Athens University Medical School in Greece, and co-author of the study. Foods high in protein, like yogurt, cheese, eggs, lean meats, or beans and legumes, proved to be the most satisfying in this study, followed by whole-grain breads and fruits and vegetables, which contain a significant amount of carbohydrates. This doesn't mean you should avoid nuts and other healthy fats altogether—a handful is still a great source of nutrients and can certainly satisfy a quick taste craving—just don't count on them to fill you up.

225 Mute the music to work more efficiently

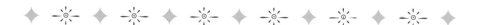

IF YOUR IDEAL WORKING environment includes your favorite tunes blaring in the background, you may be doing yourself a disservice. According to recent research from the United Kingdom, listening to music while you work—whether it's Mozart or catchy Top 40 tracks—can inhibit your performance. In the study, people were asked to memorize a series of letters. Those who tried to remember and recall the sequence while listening to music, regardless of whether it was music they liked or music they hated, had a harder time than people who did the task in silence. However, not all sound had the same effect: People who worked in what researchers called a steady-state environment, in this case, while listening to a recording of someone repeating the same word time after time, did just as well as those who worked in silence. In other words, ambient noise—like the unvarying sound that comes from a trickling water feature—is okay, but your favorite playlist is not. Other studies have shown that listening to music *before* a task can help boost performance, so if you're yearning for some tunes, hit "play" while you're prepping for a project, then pause the track when it's time to get down to business.

226 Forge friendships for better health

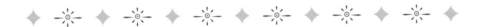

YOU KNOW THE THINGS YOU can do to improve your health: avoid cigarettes, eat mindfully, exercise regularly, and try to keep your stress levels in check, to name a few. But there's another—somewhat unexpected—behavior to add to your list of healthy habits: an active social life. According to researchers at Brigham Young University, who analyzed 148 studies on the subject, having strong connections with friends and family can actually improve your overall chances of living longer by 50 percent. In other words, a lack of social support can be just as harmful to your health as some of the more obvious risk factors, like drinking heavily.

If making friends comes naturally to you, continue to put effort into forging and maintaining bonds, particularly as you get older, which is when loneliness is more apt to set in. If you're naturally shy, you can still find ways to build your own community: join established groups like a book club, church choir, or boot-camp class to meet like-minded people, and make a little extra effort to learn about your neighbors and co-workers, too. You needn't seek out dozens of new contacts—having even a couple of close friends can improve your health.

227

Stay on track on trips

VACATIONS ARE YOUR TIME TO relax and decompress, but that doesn't have to mean derailing all the diet and exercise efforts you've made in your everyday life. According to research from the University of Copenhagen, if your activity level drops from moderate to low for as short a time as fourteen days—which could be caused by, say, lounging poolside for two weeks—you can increase your risk of diabetes, decrease your muscle mass, and lower your cardiovascular fitness by 7 percent. To get motivated while on vacation, find active ways to explore your new surroundings, such as strolls on the beach, hikes in the woods, or a bike ride on the boardwalk. You'll burn off more mojitos and feel increasingly energized, not to mention pen more exciting postcards. Plus, you may look even better after your vacation than you did before you left!

228 Tap into gratitude to get happy

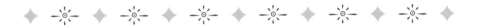

HAPPINESS COMES AND GOES, but there are ways you can keep it around longer, make it stronger, and experience it more consistently. Those are the findings of Sonja Lyubomirsky, PhD, professor of psychology at the University of California, Riverside, and author of *The How of Happiness: A Scientific Approach to Getting the Life You Want.* It turns out that happiness may not be as elusive as we once thought.

According to several of Lyubomirsky's studies, an easy way to boost mood is to focus on the daily events that make you happy, from interacting with a cheery grocery store cashier to arriving at the bus stop just in time to catch a ride. To be more aware of these events, note them in a gratitude journal, so that you notice them in the moment and reflect back on them once more when writing them down. Simply penning a few sentences about what you're grateful for can increase happiness levels, according to Lyubomirsky's research, and even subjects who expressed feelings of gratitude just once a week got a boost.

229 Your slim-down secret weapon: a bus pass

IF FEARS OF GERMS OR CROWDED cars prevent you from taking public transportation, you're doing yourself a major fitness disservice. In addition to saving you money on gas and parking, and putting less wear and tear on the environment, riding the bus, ferry, or train helps you lose weight, according to scientists. In one recent study from two Pennsylvania universities, researchers found that people who switched from driving everywhere to using a light-rail system lost an average of about six pounds in a year. The theory is that by walking the extra blocks it takes to get to and from bus stops and train stations—instead of pulling up right in front of a destination—you naturally increase your activity level enough to result in weight loss. If public transit isn't an option for you, look for other ways to add extra walking to your errand-running and commute: for example, you can park a few blocks away from your destination to increase your step count.

230 Plan ahead to lower stress

HAVE YOU EVER NOTICED THAT some mornings your commute can be refreshing, and other mornings it leaves you on edge? The same trek can affect you differently depending on how much pressure you've placed on yourself, says David Strayer, PhD, professor of psychology at The University of Utah. Take the mornings that send your stress levels rising. Chances are you're running late, which makes you drive with an increased sense of urgency, passing every vehicle you can. This competitive stress, where you jockey for the first place in line, is deeply ingrained, says Strayer, but if you trigger it—like you do when you're in a rush—your internal reaction is often great enough to raise blood pressure levels. In addition to harming your health, this type of anxiety can cause irrational behavior, like dangerous driving. To make every morning feel more leisurely, and less like a time trial for an Indy race, simply add in more travel time to account for unexpected events, says Strayer. You'll arrive on time and with less stress.

231 Get your workout timing right

NOT SURE OF THE BEST TIME TO work out? Any time, according to research from Finland. In a recent study, sports scientists found that exercisers who lifted weights in the morning made similar gains in muscle and strength as people who trained in the evening. But even if your body reacts in the same way to fitness day or night, your brain may not: poll after poll has shown that morning exercisers are more likely to stick with their fitness routines than people who work out during the afternoon or at night. Researchers theorize that this is because later in the day, it's easier to find reasons to skip a workout, such as falling behind on your to-do list or being invited out for after-work drinks. Of course, it's important that you find the time that's best for your body's own rhythms, so test different workout times and see which is most convenient for you—that's the routine you're most likely to stick with.

232 Say good-bye to sugary drinks

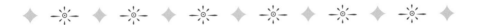

WHAT WOULD YOU GIVE TO LOSE weight without cutting out your favorite foods or adding any extra exercise to your routine? According to mounting research, the question should be, "what would you give up?"

Our drinking habits have changed drastically over the last few decades. In one recent study, Barry M. Popkin, PhD, professor of nutrition at the University of North Carolina and director of the school's Interdisciplinary Obesity Center, found that almost a quarter of the average person's calories are being slurped up through a straw, thanks to sodas, juice drinks, and other sugary beverages.

To cut calories, fill your glass with healthy beverages, says Popkin. Sparkling water can sate your carbonation craving, unsweetened coffee or tea can warm your morning, and juices made from 100 percent fruit offer lots of healthy nutrients, and many can be diluted with water to cut calories without sacrificing taste.

233 Use pressure points to perk up

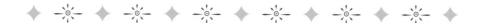

FEELING LOW ON ENERGY? IF you don't have time for a power nap, skip the coffee and energy drinks and tap into the natural recharging effects of acupressure. By stimulating the same points used in acupuncture—only with pressure, not needles—this ancient technique provides relief from hundreds of conditions with carefully guided touch, says Venus Elyse, acupuncturist and founder of Integrative Healing in Fairfax, California.

To beat fatigue, Elyse suggests using one of the most common points in Chinese medicine, Stomach-36. To locate the spot, reach down to one knee and find the bony protrusion just below and outside the joint, at the top and side of your shinbone. Measure four finger-widths down the outside of your calf and dig into the flesh about one finger-width away from your shinbone until you find a tender spot. Rather than press with force, gently massage this area as though you're polishing a stone, suggests Elyse. Rub the area for around five minutes each hour to get an energy boost and, as a bonus, you'll also ease digestive problems.

234

Spread on sunblock before fastening your seatbelt

IF YOU'RE DRIVING, DON'T COUNT on your car to protect you from sun damage. According to one recent study, co-authored by Scott W. Fosko, MD, chair of the department of dermatology at the Saint Louis University School of Medicine, more skin cancers are reported on the left side of the body than on the right, largely because of time spent in the car. In fact, malignant melanoma cases happen three times as often on the left side as on the right. No matter how you get around, you should apply sunblock each morning, and reapply it periodically throughout the day. If you spend a lot of time in your car, consider wearing long sleeves and hats while you drive, or tinting your windows with a UV-blocking film.

235 Make your own luck

BEFORE A BIG GAME OR PRESEN-
tation, do you ever knock on wood or cross
your fingers? Superstitious rituals may not
actually improve your performance, but
simply believing that they will appears to
give you a boost. That's the conclusion of
a recent German study, in which subjects
were asked to play a memory game either
with or without their lucky charm: those
who held onto their talisman actually
performed better than those who were
asked to play without it. Researchers think
that a boost in confidence brought on these
results—people who believe deeply in their
own superstitions are convinced they'll
perform better when they hold that lucky
charm or perform that ritual, and this con-
viction becomes a self-fulfilling prophecy.
So, while that rabbit's foot may not have
inherently magical powers, if you think it
does, keep using it.

236 Steer clear of decision-making during mood extremes

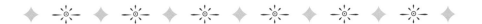

IF YOU'VE EVER DOWNED A PINT of ice cream after a breakup—or over-indulged in something else after a difficult experience—it should come as no surprise that feeling overwhelmed, stressed, or negative can lead to less self-control. What you may not know is that this same sort of spontaneous behavior accompanies excitement, too. According to Vanessa M. Patrick, PhD, associate professor at the University of Houston's C.T. Bauer College of Business, feeling giddy—like after getting a promotion at work, or winning a fierce game of tennis—can also lead to lapses in judgment.

No doubt you've experienced this—just think back on your last celebratory indulgence, like a happy hour or shopping spree. These occasions don't necessarily snowball into permanent bad habits, but it's important to recognize that how you're feeling can shape your choices, particularly if you're going through an unusually positive or negative period, says Patrick. If you're trying to reach a goal—like saving money—you may need to muster up more self-control when you're feeling particularly high or low. If your emotions are jumping around a lot, try to save big decisions for when you're in a more stable mood.

237

Tune out the static and increase your focus

IN THIS LOGGED-ON, PLUGGED-IN world, it's standard to have your attention and energy drawn in dozens of directions at once. The downside of this information overload is that it can make focusing extremely difficult. To increase your attention span as well as enhance your ability to notice details, try meditation. According to one recent study from the University of California, Davis, an intense Buddhist meditation practice helped participants increase their ability to focus on a task, even if the task was boring. The idea is that meditation—sitting still and in silence while observing your thoughts—helps train people to engage in other less stimulating activities. The amount of meditation training employed by this study was quite high—five hours a day over a three-month period—but smaller amounts can help you to slow down and focus, too.

238 Shop healthy for yourself and others

IF YOU'RE IN CHARGE OF GROCERY shopping for others—whether you stock your family's kitchen every week or are just picking up munchies for a party—you may be unwittingly sabotaging their attempts at staying healthy: researchers from the University of Miami found that people made healthier choices when selecting foods just for themselves than when they were picking out foods for other people. If you tend to buy veggies and fruits for *your* meals, but splurge on cookies and chips when you're buying for your loved ones, swap out a few indulgent foods for healthier options. You'll spread around the wellness benefits.

239

Set goals to stave off Alzheimer's

AS YOU CHECK THINGS OFF YOUR life to-do list, be sure you keep adding new goals, particularly as you age. A new study on Alzheimer's disease found that older adults who felt the greatest sense of purpose—such as a cause they actively promoted, family who relied on them, or a local organization they were involved with—were less likely to develop the disease. In fact, according to researchers from Rush University Medical Center in Chicago, who analyzed 951 people for the study, seniors who were still engaged and working toward goals reduced their risk of developing Alzheimer's disease by 52 percent. Even if you're too young to worry about the condition yourself, strive to help older relatives, friends, and community members develop goals and direction in their lives to help them maintain healthy minds for years to come.

240 Focus your language to fight fair

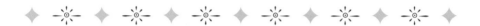

WHEN YOU FIND YOURSELF IN A disagreement, choose your words carefully. "When emotions come in to play, which is often the case when conflicts happen, the most natural response is blame, which starts with 'you did,' 'you always,' or 'you never,'" says Lynne Hurdle-Price, president of Hurdle-Price Professionals, a conflict resolution and diversity awareness consulting organization. "When the other person hears this, it almost automatically puts them on the defensive—they feel as though they're being called the bad guy."

Hurdle-Price suggests speaking in sentences that start with "I" so that you express your feelings without assigning blame. "When 'you' statements are used, often the only word the other person hears is 'you,' 'you,' 'you.' If you use an 'I' statement, you are not blaming them, you are stating your feelings and the reason for your feelings and expressing and hoping for a potential solution."

"I" statements can be hard to make, says Hurdle-Price. They don't always feel natural in the moment, so if possible, practice them ahead of time to make sure that what you're saying is what you want the other person to hear. Then, sit back and listen. "'I' statements are best followed up by some good active listening to the other person's response and then another 'I' statement in response to them if necessary."

241

Learn to spot fats in your snacks

IN ORDER TO EAT NUTRITIOUSLY, you don't need to avoid all processed food: plenty of healthy choices come pre-packaged, such as certain yogurts and cereals. But learning the right way to look at a food's ingredients list can aid your healthy eating pursuits, says Bonnie Taub-Dix, MA, RD, CDN, author of *Read It Before You Eat It*, a book that helps make sense of food nutrition labels.

Ingredients lists are written in descending order, from the item that's used most in a food down through the item that's used the least. Use this placement to determine just how healthy a food is. For example, if you're eating multigrain bread, you want 100 percent whole wheat to be first on the list, or at least in the top three, says Taub-Dix. And, if you're having canned peaches or pears, you don't want to see high-fructose corn syrup and sugar listed before the fruit. If it is, you're getting a big bite of sugar and calories, and very little in the way of nutrients or vitamins.

242

Pitch in at local parks

IF YOU ENJOY SPENDING TIME outdoors, consider volunteering at a nearby park or preserve. According to a study co-authored by Rachel Kaplan, PhD, professor of environment and behavior at the University of Michigan, the benefits of spending time in nature are the same whether you're outside for recreation or to work. But when volunteering outdoors, you'll improve not just your state of mind, but the environment itself.

Volunteering can provide the chance to meet others, learn new skills, make a difference, contribute to your community, and feel connected to the environment. You can find hundreds of Web sites that match people with volunteer opportunities, and local parks and recreation departments are always in need of help.

243 Practice resting to sleep better

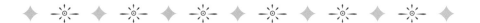

YOU MAY THINK OF SLEEP PREP- aration as those five minutes you spend brushing your teeth, washing your face, and changing into your pajamas before bed. But according to John Friend, founder of Anusara yoga, a style of yoga now practiced in seventy countries, most people could use a nighttime ritual readjustment.

Focusing on your breath at bedtime can help you to fall into a deep slumber. But if minding your inhales and exhales isn't helping you to fall asleep, try focusing on your breathing throughout the day. "If

your sympathetic system doesn't know how to relax, particularly after a stressful day, or a scary experience, you're going to toss and turn," says Friend.

To unwind, practice makes perfect. You can help train your body to relax when you want it to by pausing throughout your day and taking about three minutes to focus on your breath, suggests Friend. By strengthening your calm response when you're in the midst of a stressful situation, you'll find it easier to detach when it's time to rest and recharge.

244 Get S.M.A.R.T. about workout goals

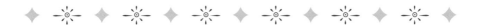

IF YOU'VE PACKED ON THE pounds over the years, nothing says that you can't one day reach your dream weight with the right combination of fitness and diet, but big changes take time. To set goals that keep you motivated for the long haul, you have to be S.M.A.R.T., says Gerald K. Endress, MS, fitness director of the Duke University Diet and Fitness Center. Here's how:

FIRST, MAKE GOALS SPECIFIC: Want to lose weight? Great! Figure out how many pounds you're over and set a goal of losing that exact amount.

THEN, FIND A WAY TO MEASURE YOUR PROGRESS: To track if you've lost weight, you'll need a scale. This way you can celebrate victories and know when to work a bit harder.

NEXT, BE SURE IT'S ATTAINABLE: If you're expecting to look like a runway model, reconsider what weight is going to make you happy and healthy.

THAT'S WHERE BEING REALISTIC COMES IN: In order to lose weight, what changes are you willing to make? How much you're willing to work will determine if a goal is not only doable, but likely.

FINALLY, YOUR GOAL SHOULD BE TIMELY: A year-long goal—like losing fifty pounds in twelve months—may seem like a good idea, but setting mini-goals can help you to stay motivated. Backtrack from your ultimate dream so you can check off milestones along the way.

245

Out of sight, out of mind to heal a broken heart

AFTER A BAD BREAKUP OR AN unexpected layoff, you know that the healthiest thing to do is to move on, but that's easier said than done. How exactly do you put the past behind you when you're trying to recover from an emotionally taxing experience? According to researchers at the University of Toronto, physically packing away mementos and reminders of the painful experience can help give you the traction you need to move forward. Based on their findings, it's nearly impossible to simply turn off your feelings, but removing tangible reminders of bad memories—actively sealing them away in a closed box and putting them out of sight—seems to help people let go of the past. Pictures, gifts, and even old journals are fair game—just note what no longer makes you feel good and pack it away.

246

Stretch away muscle soreness

WHEN YOU WORK OUT AT YOUR max—pushing yourself to lift a little harder or run a little faster than you think you can—you actually cause small tears in your muscle. When these tears heal, you get stronger, but in the meantime, they can cause some pretty noticeable discomfort. This pain, called delayed onset muscle soreness, typically shows up twenty-four to forty-eight hours after a tough workout and can last for several days. Studies show that light activity such as stretching or walking can help to ease tender areas, and by increasing blood flow to those muscles, you may speed up your recovery, too. If you're sore after a hard workout, head out for a slow to moderate walk around the block and do a few gentle stretches when you return. Even this small amount of activity will help ease aches.

247 Communication takes more than just talk

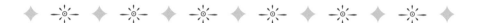

WHEN YOU ENTER A DISCUSSION, you may think that the speaker holds the power. After all, that's the person whom all eyes and ears are trained on. But according to Susanne Conrad, a communications advisor who has helped companies around the world improve interpersonal and business relations, it's actually the listeners who hold the cards.

"A person can talk as much as they want, but if you aren't listening, or if your listening is clouded by your internal dialogue, then you actually take all of the power out of their words," says Conrad. When another person starts to talk, try to remain objective as you listen to his or her words. If you don't

agree with what this person is saying, don't shut down your hearing and start forming a rebuttal; if a friend is telling you about his problem don't begin to think about how what he's saying will affect you; and if you hear news you don't like, try not to block it out with thoughts like, "Of course this is what's happening" or "Oh well."

Just listen. Only when you open your ears and your heart and hear what another person is actually saying will you really communicate, says Conrad. Until then, what you think of as a conversation is likely just a couple of monologues running together side by side.

248 Steer clear of body blues

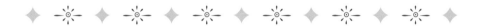

FLIPPING THROUGH A MAGAZINE is supposed to be a pleasant pastime, but it can actually make you feel worse. What gives? According to Heather Hausenblas, PhD, associate professor of applied physiology and kinesiology at the University of Florida, looking at pictures of the "ideal physique" as presented in the media has a negative effect on people.

"After seeing pictures of models in media, such as in magazines and on billboards and TV, people report that they are more body dissatisfied, in a worse mood, and more depressed, anxious, and angry," says Hausenblas. And while the negative effects of media on women have been widely reported, men are just as susceptible.

Some brands have embraced the idea of using real people in their campaigns, but the trend hasn't entirely caught on. In the meantime, Hausenblas suggests taking in images with a grain of salt. "What you see isn't real," says Hausenblas. "Keep in mind that models represent a small fraction of the population, and almost every image has been retouched and altered." In other words, these pictures don't represent reality. Remembering this may help you be less judgmental about your own body. But if you start to feel down, walk it off: according to Hausenblas's other research, exercise of any sort is one surefire way to boost your own body image.

249 Use peppermint to put pep back in your step

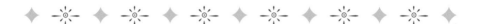

EVEN IF YOU START YOUR DAY ultra-energized and with the best of intentions, chances are that you may begin to have trouble focusing sometime around 3 p.m.—something office workers everywhere call the afternoon slump. Unfortunately, most employers don't encourage after-lunch siestas. But there are ways to get back on track without taking a power nap. To help stimulate your senses and snap back your focus, take a whiff of peppermint essential oil, suggests Hope Gillerman, a holistic healer and creator of a line of essential oil–based remedies and care products.

In her aromatherapy practice, Gillerman prescribes peppermint essential oil to clients who need a bit of mental clarity. A single whiff of the oil stimulates the body and focuses the mind for a couple of hours. To keep the clarifying properties with you for longer, dilute the essential oil in an unscented carrier oil—such as jojoba oil—and rub it on your neck and shoulders when your focus starts to fade. You can also scent a room with the oil: simply put a few drops on a tissue and place it on your desk and let the smell slowly fill your office.

250 When it's okay to imagine the worst

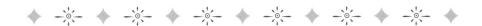

YOU'VE HEARD ABOUT POSITIVE visualizations—where you imagine the best possible outcome in a situation and actually see yourself achieving those results. But in some circumstances, it's helpful to imagine the worst-case scenario instead. This sort of negative visualization, says Andrew Taggart, PhD, a philosophical counselor in New York City, can help you to prepare for unexpected events.

Take, for example, riding your bike to run errands, explains Taggart. Rather than simply jumping on your bike and riding off, spend a moment imagining both the expected and unexpected things that might happen to you—passing cars may be going too fast, a car door could swing open in your path, or a pedestrian might dart out in front of you. Because you've imagined these somewhat jarring circumstances beforehand, you're actually better prepared to handle whatever comes your way when you're actually riding, says Taggart.

In addition, negative visualization will also help you to stay present. When biking, you'll be less reactive when a car honks its horn and may appreciate the whole experience more. This process can be applied to all areas of your life, and may also stir up extra appreciation. For example, if you were to imagine a negative emotional experience, such as the loss of a loved one, you'd immediately be reminded of how important that person is to you and act accordingly.

251

Deter dementia with higher education

IF YOU'RE TRYING TO DECIDE whether or not you should go back to school, European researchers have a new item to add to your pro-school list: the more education you receive, the lower your chances of developing dementia later in life. In the study, which examined the brains of 872 people, scientists found that for each year of education you accumulate, you reduce your risk of suffering from dementia by 11 percent. The connection between school and brain function remains unclear, but scientists suspect that rather than protecting the brain from the condition, education somehow makes the brain better able to compensate for changes brought on by dementia and keeps the symptoms at bay. Other effective ways to stave off dementia include eating a diet that's high in nutrients and omega-3 fats, exercising regularly, and getting enough vitamin D.

252 Drink your way to a better workout

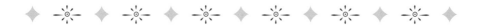

FORGET ABOUT FANCY SPORTS drinks: most come loaded with sugar and some lack the nutrients you need to replenish your system after a long workout. Water can help you to stay hydrated, and recent studies show that some of the best drinks for burning fat and building muscle may be the ones you're already drinking.

If you're strength training, drink a glass of milk after a session of weight lifting to help you build more muscle and boost bone health thanks to the presence of protein, fat, and calcium. If cardio training is your thing, try drinking several cups of green tea each day, which studies show helps your body burn more fat during exercise by speeding up your metabolism. And don't forget coffee. A number of studies have highlighted the benefits of drinking a cup of joe: it provides extra energy and endurance, it reduces pain, and according to some research, it may even contribute to enhanced sun protection during a workout.

253 The downside of overanalyzing your problems

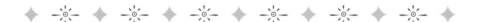

IF YOU'RE GOING THROUGH A tough time, your first instinct may be to sit down with a friend and tell him or her all about it. That's okay up to a point, says Amanda Rose, PhD, associate professor in the University of Missouri department of psychological sciences. But rehashing the same event over and over again can actually cause you to get more upset, not less.

"Talking about problems isn't necessarily counterproductive," says Rose, "but the rehashing of details, speculating about the situation, and talking about sad feelings over and over is." This sort of behavior usually won't make you feel better, and will often leave you feeling worse than before. To keep your conversation in check, allow yourself enough time to air your grievances to a friend once—for, say, twenty minutes— then switch your banter to other subjects. Rather than just vent, make some of that time productive by steering the conversation toward problem solving and what you can do to feel better so that your talk has a positive aspect.

254 Decompress during your commute

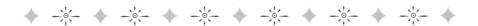

WHETHER IT TAKES YOU MINUTES or hours to get home from the office, all work-related thoughts should be history by the time you step in the front door, says Gabriela Corá, MD, MBA, founder of the Executive Health & Wealth Institute in Miami, Florida. To ease the transition from work to home, make the most of your drive, walk, or subway ride.

"If you're still on the phone and checking e-mails after you leave work, your commute is just an extension of your day at the office," explains Corá. To arrive home fresh, shift your attention away from your job. If you're driving a car, listen to music, a comedy show, or an audio book to divert your thoughts; if you're riding a train or bus, read an enjoyable book or play games on your mobile phone.

According to Corá, some people may be able to make the shift from work mode to the rest of their lives very quickly, but most of us require a fifteen- to thirty-minute break. It may mean setting strict boundaries—like vowing not to check e-mail until you're back in the office—but it's worth it. Taking the time you need to transition from office to home will help you to walk into your house refreshed and ready to enjoy your non-work hours.

255 Never be without a goal

WHEN YOU REACH A GOAL, GO ahead and savor your success—but don't linger too long on your current achievements. In order to continue reaching more and bigger goals, you need to focus on the future, says Ayelet Fishbach, PhD, professor of behavioral science and marketing at the University of Chicago Booth School of Business.

"Focusing on attainable future goals makes people want to achieve more and increase their level of engagement and aspiration," says Fishbach, who studies goal-setting. So, if you just nailed a work presentation, revel in the glory for a bit, then set a new goal for yourself, such as attracting a certain amount of new business, or completing a management class. Writing down goals, then checking them off as you meet them, can help you keep track of all you've accomplished, as well as all that you still have yet to achieve.

256 Expand your approach to recycling

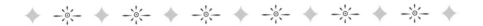

WHEN IT COMES TO YOUR JUNK, think outside the recycling bin. You probably have bins to separate plastic, metal, glass, and paper, but those are only some of the everyday items you can dispose of in a green way, says Jennifer Schwab, LEED AP, director of sustainability for Sierra Club Green Home, an organization that helps people to green their living space. Reusing, repurposing, and safely disposing of goods can keep landfills from filling up and ensure that harmful toxins don't make it into the heap.

Batteries, printer cartridges, appliances, and paints are only a few of the items that shouldn't be dumped in with your trash,

says Schwab. To learn your options, search online for local recycling centers, or return to the store where you purchased an item to ask about proper disposal. Oftentimes, electronics like cell phones, computers, and TVs can be used for parts or refurbished and resold, so big box stores frequently accept them. The same goes for old appliances like blenders and refrigerators. If your possessions are still in working order, consider donating them: second-hand stores will often accept household goods as well as shoes, clothing, and furniture, which can extend their use and keep them out of the garbage pile.

257 Turn off the TV to take off pounds

IF YOU WANT TO LOSE WEIGHT but are having a hard time sticking to a low-calorie diet or regular exercise plan, switching off the television may be all that you need to get your health back on track. In one study out of The University of Vermont, thirty-six couch potatoes were asked to cut their TV time in half: this simple change in routine helped people burn an extra 119 calories each day without even trying. The idea is that less time spent sitting in front of the tube will equal more time doing other everyday activities, such as cleaning the house, going for a stroll after dinner, or participating in a hobby like cooking. All of this extra motion zaps calories, and by limiting television, you'll reclaim valuable hours in your day, too.

258 Use conversational cues to curb rambling

YOU ALWAYS NOTICE WHEN someone else starts to ramble on, but it's not so easy to pick up on your own long-winded tendencies. When you're telling a story, answering a question, or giving a presentation, it can be hard to tell if you've gotten off topic or gone on for too long. After all, most people will try to suppress a yawn while you're speaking, even if they're feeling bored. But here's one telltale sign that your audience's attention is waning: they increase the number of times they blink their eyes. According to researchers at the University of Waterloo in Canada, people blink twice as frequently—increasing from around ten blinks per minute to twenty—when their minds have wandered. So if you notice an associate's lashes start to flutter, wrap up your chatter. Or, if you're the one whose mind is starting to wander, try to bring your focus back to the person who's talking.

259 Power your movements with breath

BREATH IS EMPHASIZED IN PILATES work, but all of that inhaling and exhaling at certain times may seem a bit arbitrary—in class, your mind may be working so hard to move your arms and legs that simply breathing is enough of a challenge. Pilates is based on the principle of exhaling during exertion, when the move becomes most difficult, and inhaling as a preparation, or cleaning of the slate, says Alycea Ungaro, owner of Real Pilates, a fitness center in New York, and author of the *Pilates Practice Companion*. And, just as this breath pattern can help during traditional Pilates moves, it can also be applied to your everyday life. Just think about some of the things you do regularly—hefting bags of groceries or giving presentations to your colleagues, for example. "Pilates trains you to use your breath as a tool instinctively," says Ungaro. Inhale to welcome new challenges, then exhale to get ready for some heavy lifting.

260 "Organic" isn't everything

DON'T FALL PREY TO THE
common misconception that eating organic
gives you a free pass to stop counting
calories. In a recent study out of Cornell
University, scientists found that people who
ate a cookie labeled "organic" estimated that
it contained 40 percent fewer calories than
a label-free cookie. Surprise: the cookies
were identical. While organic foods may
contain fewer chemicals than their non-
organic counterparts, they're not necessarily
healthier choices in terms of fat and calorie
content. To make the best decisions for
your body, read the entire label, not just the
"organic" tag.

261 Fitness fix: don't forget your feet

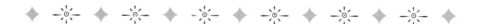

YOUR FEET ARE VITAL FOR walking and staying balanced, which means they work hard all day long. But when's the last time you gave these overtaxed body parts a little TLC? To ease aches and relax cramped feet, all you need is a small rubber ball, says Sue Hitzmann, founder of Longevity Fitness Inc. and creator of the M.E.L.T. Method, a type of self-massage that uses props like the ball and long, cylindrical foam rollers.

To start, place the rubber ball—which should have a diameter of about ¾ inch/ 2 centimeters—on the ground. Set one foot on the ball so the ball is under the center of the foot, heel on the floor. Flex and curl your toes like opening and closing a fist, then wiggle them, all while applying light to moderate pressure to the ball. Next, lift your foot and lightly press down on the ball just below your big toe joint. Roll the ball from toe to heel, applying light pressure. Lift your foot and reposition the ball under your second toe joint and repeat, rolling from each toe down to the heel in what Hitzmann calls a rinsing pattern. Finally, quickly move your foot front, back, and side over the ball—almost like you're shaking your foot—pressing down moderately and pausing to circle around any tender areas. Repeat on your other foot.

262

The benefits of saying thank you

DON'T LET GOOD DEEDS GO un-thanked. According to research done by Christopher Peterson, PhD, psychology professor at the University of Michigan, saying thank you can lead to an improved mood.

In one study, Peterson asked subjects to think of a person who had made an impact on their life but never been properly thanked. Those subjects wrote a letter of gratitude to that person, then hand-delivered the note and talked about what they had written. The letter writers felt good in the moment and reported a boost in mood for the next month.

Putting in place a regular ritual of giving thanks can make you more aware of all you have to be grateful for, and also help you to build bonds with the people you value most in your life. Reflect on the ways in which others have touched your life, from influential teachers to helpful neighbors and friends. As regularly as you can, recognize those people with a note of thanks.

263 Ease shoulder tension in two minutes

WHEN YOU'RE FEELING STRESSED, your neck and shoulders may start to ache. But this sort of soreness can be avoided. "Shoulder tension is often due to head placement," says Joan Arnold, a certified teacher of the Alexander Technique in New York City. As you lift your shoulders from stress, your head starts to fall back, taking your body out of alignment. By relaxing and lengthening the neck, you'll be able to soften the shoulders and bring the head back to a more comfortable position.

When you start to feel tense, close your eyes for two minutes and think about your neck as an open channel for breath, suggests Arnold. This helps your head move into a place where it's balanced atop your spine with a slight tilt forward—a position that allows your neck and shoulders to relax and air to pass through with ease. Keep this position in mind throughout your day; make time for a quick posture check each time you start to feel tense.

264 Hit the hiking trail for an exciting workout

IF YOU WANT TO STAY FIT BUT can't stand the tedium of the gym, consider hiking your workout windfall. Head out for a day hike with friends, and the spectacular views will distract you from your physical exertion. But don't be fooled: the changes in terrain during a hike make for an interval workout that targets your entire lower body.

A note of caution: steep slopes can do a number on tender knees, so if you ever experience knee pain, invest in a pair of walking poles. Research from Austria has found that they relieve pressure on the knee joints by about 25 percent, which means less wear and tear. And as a bonus, using trekking poles can increase your calorie burn without making the workout feel more difficult, according to researchers at James Madison University.

265 Learn a language to boost your memory

VAMOS! ALLER! VAS-Y! IF YOU'VE always meant to learn a second—or third, or fourth—language, stop stalling and order those Spanish CDs or enroll in that French class: new research shows that being able to speak, read, or write more than one language actually enhances memory. What's more, a recent study shows that people who are multilingual appear to have an easier time solving complex problems, which has led the Finnish scientists behind the study to theorize that knowing more than one language boosts other cognitive skills, too. Best of all, this increase in brainpower occurs long before you reach fluency: simply starting to learn a new tongue can increase your brainpower.

266 The anticancer diet

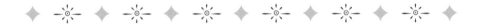

YOU *CAN* EAT TO PREVENT CANCER, but the secret isn't in stocking up on a single ingredient. Though clinical trials have been performed on hundreds of foods, including raspberries, kale, green tea, nuts, and spices like turmeric, no true superfood has been found to keep cancer at bay. Instead, more balanced eating habits seem to be the most effective way to prevent cancer.

"Of all of the foods and nutrients—including supplements—that have been studied over many years, the only thing that has really proven to have a major impact on many cancers is obesity," says Nancy Cotugna, DrPH, RD, professor of nutrition at the University of Delaware. The American Cancer Institute supports this, maintaining that keeping the body at a healthy weight is one of the most important things a person can do to reduce his or her risk of cancer.

"The best dietary advice for lowering cancer risk is to eat more fruits, vegetables, whole grains, and legume-type beans, and to eat less red and processed meats and avoid alcohol, or at least limit it to no more than one drink a day for women and two for men," says Cotugna. Also on the list: choosing mainly plant-based foods as part of your diet and getting thirty minutes or more of physical activity every day. By aiming to do all of these, you'll best protect your body.

267

Alleviate major worries by working out

IF YOU'RE A BORN WORRYWART, you may find that your anxiety gets the best of you at times. But there's a natural way to relieve some of your fears: studies have shown that aerobic exercise can ease mild anxiety, and according to recent research by Rodney K. Dishman, PhD, professor of exercise science at the University of Georgia, regular physical activity can temper severe anxiety, too.

Exactly how exercise helps to reduce or eliminate major anxiety—such as the onset of panic attacks—remains unclear, says Dishman. People may start to worry less because they're doing something positive for themselves, because of the distraction exercise provides, or due to a physical reaction, such as the release of endorphins. Whatever the cause, Dishman recommends aiming for 150 minutes of moderate-intensity activity or 75 minutes of vigorous working out per week to help alleviate anxiety. More is probably better, says Dishman, but less is better than nothing.

268 Fill up on fiber

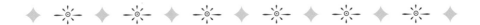

SWAPPING OUT A FEW ITEMS IN your fridge or pantry may be all it takes to start losing weight. But don't simply replace your high-fat and high-calorie snacks with light versions—a lot of so-called diet foods aren't very filling, which means you eat more to stay satisfied, increasing your calorie count along the way. Instead, stock your kitchen with fiber-rich foods.

"A high-fiber diet, such as one that includes whole grains, vegetables, legumes, and fruits, should be included in any weight-loss diet," says Lalita Kaul, PhD, RD, LDN, ADA spokesperson, professor at Howard University's College of Medicine. Fiber expands in your stomach, and takes a significant amount of time to digest, which makes it a good choice for anyone who wants to limit snacking or stay full on smaller portions. Adults should eat between 25 and 38 grams of fiber each day. But don't go overboard. While more fiber may sound like a good idea, it's not—eating more than the recommended amount can result in stomach pains and may even obstruct the digestive tract.

269

The surprise supplement for building better bones

CALCIUM CONSUMPTION CAN improve bone health. But on its own, the calcium in foods and supplements isn't always absorbed. In order to benefit from the bone-building properties of this nutrient, you also need to increase your intake of vitamin D, says Hector DeLuca, PhD, the biochemistry department chair at the University of Wisconsin-Madison.

"There's no doubt about the importance of vitamin D to bone health," says DeLuca. "If you're vitamin D deficient you're not going to absorb calcium." Sunblock blocks most of the vitamin D we could absorb naturally from the sun, and the nutrient is not commonly found in foods, so taking a supplement is generally recommended. To maximize your bone health, take a supplement that has both calcium and vitamin D. If you're unsure about the proper dosage, check with your doctor.

270

Amp up your sex life by working your pelvic floor

YOU'VE HEARD WOMEN PROCLAIM that Kegel exercises are the secret to better sex, and the pelvic floor–strengthening squeezes work for men, too: one recent study found that Kegels helped to improve men's stamina and gave them stronger erections. To perform a Kegel, practice contracting your pelvic floor muscles—the ones you use to stop urination. The squeezes can be done anywhere—seated, standing, or lying down—just aim to hold each contraction for a few seconds, then repeat, increasing your number of reps as you go. For a full-body workout with Kegel-like effects, try Pilates. This style of core-strengthening exercise provides a real workout for the pelvic floor.

271 Get your focus back, fast

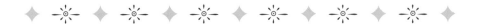

IF YOUR FOCUS IS FADING, GIVE into the urge to walk away from your work: one recent study found that taking a stroll in nature can boost short-term memory and attention span by 20 percent. Sure, exercise is invigorating, but what makes this trick actually work is that you're shifting from one type of attention to another, says Marc Berman, PhD, a cognitive neuroscientist at the University of Michigan and co-author of the study.

There are two types of attention, says Berman: directed attention, where you have to direct yourself to focus on something specific, like a form you're filling out; and involuntary attention, where something automatically holds your focus, like a waterfall or a beautiful painting.

You have limited stores of directed attention, but switching to an activity that requires only involuntary attention can help you to get your focus back. In the study, walking in nature for fifty minutes produced the same attention and memory boost as viewing photographs of nature, but walking along city streets didn't improve memory or attention. The reason: an urban setting full of cars and pedestrians can require a large amount of directed attention.

When you're feeling distracted and taxed, move away from the space you're working in, suggests Berman, and look for an activity that allows your mind to drift.

272

Pick protein to lose fat and keep muscle

IF YOUR WEIGHT-LOSS PLANS include cutting calories and adding exercise—as most do—a protein-rich diet can help you hang onto lean muscle mass while dropping pounds, say European researchers. In one recent study, two diets were compared, one made up of 15 percent protein, the other of 35 percent protein. The people who consumed the low-protein diet dropped more pounds overall, but a lot of what they lost was lean muscle. The high-protein group didn't lose as much weight, but they shed an equal amount of fat while maintaining that oh-so-important muscle tissue. By loading up on lean meats, fish, and dairy, while maintaining a consistent exercise routine and reduced-calorie diet, you'll see losses on the scale without sacrificing your strength.

273 Savor your surroundings

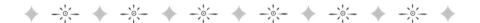

WHEN YOU'RE CAUGHT UP IN AN internal recitation of anxieties and never-ending to-do lists, it's easy to feel trapped in a ceaseless cycle of stress. But turning down the volume on your mental chatter and becoming more present isn't as difficult as you may think, says Linda Lantieri, director of The Inner Resilience Program, an organization focused on building emotional strength in school teachers. All it takes is a little training to learn to live in the moment.

To get started, try this: Each time you walk somewhere—to the office break room, to your car, to a friend's house—quiet your internal dialogue and instead pay attention to your surroundings. Focus on the smells in the air, the colors you see, the sounds you hear—just be where you are, right in that moment.

"By walking with a more present awareness, you get to wherever you're going in the same amount of time, but you arrive with a completely different state of mind," says Lantieri. By choosing to focus on just one thing—in this case, walking to your destination—you'll strengthen your ability to shift from what's happening in your mind to what's happening around you. This break from stress-inducing inner dialogue not only strengthens your mind, says Lantieri, it also nourishes your soul.

274 Root yourself with root vegetables

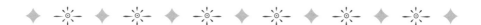

NO DOUBT YOU'VE EXPERIENCED moments when you felt like you weren't in control of your life—during periods of transition or uncertainty, or when you were simply moving so fast you couldn't keep up. In times like these, it's wise to take a page from Ayurvedic medicine, suggests holistic health counselor Amanda Misrac. According to this practice, root vegetables are incredibly grounding, making them good to eat when you're feeling a little untethered.

"Root vegetables grow deep in the earth in a quiet state that seems almost meditative," says Misrac. Much of our food grows above ground, in direct contact with the sun, wind, and rain; in the Ayurvedic tradition, roots are thought to have a calmer energy. "It seems so natural that food coming from deep in the soil can literally bring us back down to earth and keep us grounded," says Misrac. To restore feelings of stability, explore cooking with radishes, beets, parsnips, rutabaga, and sweet potatoes, all of which grow in the ground. Of course, if you feel too deeply rooted, or want to feel more prepared for change, start eating "freer" foods, like leafy vegetables, which can help you feel less bound.

275 Get smarter while you sleep

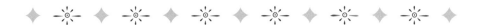

PEOPLE HAVE PROBABLY TOLD you to "just sleep on it" when you're trying to work through a problem or make a big decision, like whether or not to take a new job you've been offered. And, while it may sound like a good way to stop thinking about the issue for a bit, the act of sleeping can actually help you find the solutions you're searching for, according to the latest research from Beth Israel Deaconess Medical Center, a teaching hospital for Harvard Medical School. In a recent study, people were asked to try to solve a tricky puzzle, and afterward spent ninety minutes either napping or doing other quiet activities. Following the break, they attempted the puzzle again: The people who stayed awake showed no improvement in ability, but the sleepers who didn't dream showed small gains. However, the group who had dreamed about the puzzle improved up to 10 percent after sleeping. Scientists theorize that these results may be dependent on how much difficulty a person has with the problem; of those who were allowed to sleep, the ones who dreamed about the puzzle had been initially the worst at solving it, and their struggles with the problem may have inspired the dreams. Of course, there's no way to direct yourself to dream about a particular quandary, but if you're stuck, try going to sleep. Even if you don't dream, waking up refreshed may make you feel more ready to give it another shot!

276 Fitness fix: walk faster

IT PAYS TO PICK UP YOUR PACE, even when you're not walking for fitness. A recent study from New Zealand shows that individuals who strolled along at a window-shopping pace—around two miles per hour—for ten thousand steps burned 153 fewer calories than walkers who covered the same ground at four miles per hour. And, traveling this distance—about five miles—took thirty minutes longer for the slow strollers. Of course, there's a time to walk with less vigor—like when you really *are* window shopping, or you want to take a leisurely stroll with a friend—but if you're running errands or fitness walking, be mindful of your pace. Increasing your speed could help you lose weight without adding distance to your walk, and you'll actually save time. To gauge your speed and intensity, take the talking test: for most of us, a four-miles-per-hour walk would make us need to take a breath after every couple of words.

277 Keep your cool during conflict

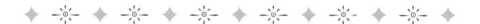

WHEN YOU'RE IN THE MIDST OF an argument—particularly one that involves someone reading off a laundry list of complaints against you—it may take all the strength you can muster just to keep your cool. But, it is possible to remain objective, even under tense circumstances. Using a few specific conflict resolution skills can help, says Lynne Hurdle-Price, president of Hurdle-Price Professionals, a conflict resolution and diversity awareness consulting organization.

"It can be very difficult to listen to someone list all of your faults or failures that led to a particular conflict," says Hurdle-Price. "But if you really stay open to listening to them and probing deeper for how they view the situation, you often find that it is not really an attack on you but rather an emotional release for them." Of course, it's hard to keep this from feeling like an ambush, but if you're able to sit back and listen, then comment on the feelings and ideas she brings up, you'll be better able to set the stage for actual discussion. To resist the urge to react with hurt feelings, remind yourself that it's important to allow another person to feel heard, and that the more you're able to learn about the other person's view, the easier it is to address the actual conflict. Feel free to respond with your own viewpoints; just try to do so in a calm, constructive way in order to move the conversation forward.

278 Skip corn syrup to slim down

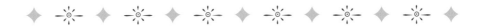

IF YOU HAVE A SWEET TOOTH, you may already be watching your calories and seeking out sugar-free replacements for your favorite snacks and drinks. But foods and beverages made with high-fructose corn syrup may actually be worse for your waistline than products that use other types of sweeteners: new research has shown that high-fructose corn syrup—one of the main ingredients in soda—can actually cause more weight gain than other sweeteners.

In an experiment performed by Bart Hoebel, PhD, professor of psychology at Princeton University, rats that drank beverages made with high-fructose corn syrup gained more weight than those drinking sugar-sweetened drinks, even though the high-fructose corn syrup drinks had fewer calories. Worst of all: the percentage of high-fructose corn syrup in the study drink was less than the amount found in a typical soft drink.

"In the six-month experiment, rats drinking high-fructose corn syrup showed greater body weight, elevated triglycerides, and heavier fat pads in the abdomen," says Hoebel. Studies are underway to determine whether the same effects will be found in humans, and to further understand how exactly high-fructose corn syrup has such an exaggerated effect on weight gain. But in the meantime, avoid food and drinks that contain high-fructose corn syrup. In addition to soda, scan the labels of drinks that aren't 100 percent fruit juice, as well as other staples, like salad dressings, soups, yogurts, and even breads and cookies.

279 Write your destiny

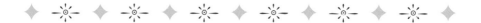

MOST OF US HAVE A GENERAL idea of the life we'd like to lead someday, but research shows that getting specific about future hopes can actually increase happiness today. Those were the findings in one study co-authored by Sonja Lyubomirsky, PhD, professor of psychology at the University of California, Riverside, and author of *The How of Happiness: A Scientific Approach to Getting the Life You Want*. When subjects were asked to detail their ideal future, their happiness levels increased dramatically.

To write your way into happiness, just grab a pen. Fantasize about your future life—where you live, what you do for work and for fun, and whom you surround yourself with. Don't be afraid to get specific: try to imagine how a typical day in this life would look and feel. Cross out, erase, and expand your ideas over time as your picture becomes clearer.

Imagining all of these future possibilities helps people sort through desires, create goals, and examine their potentials, all of which affect levels of happiness. As you learn more about yourself, you'll re-prioritize, define a greater sense of purpose, and ultimately feel more in control of your life and happiness.

280

Flu shots fight off more than a bug

A RECENT STUDY HAS FOUND that the common flu vaccine does double duty: according to scientists in the United Kingdom, in addition to reducing risk for catching a bug, these annual shots can lower your chances of having a heart attack, too. In the study, which tracked data from nearly 80,000 people, researchers found that getting a seasonal flu shot lowered a person's chance of having a heart attack by 19 percent and, if he or she got the vaccine early in the season—between September and mid-November—risk dropped even more. The scientists are unsure of the exact connection between flu shots and heart problems, but these finding suggest that the benefits of getting a shot are well worth the momentary discomfort.

281 The secret to being more efficient and effective

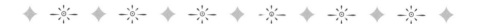

IF YOU LIKE TO JUGGLE MULTIPLE tasks at once—for example, talking on the phone, reading e-mails, and flipping through a magazine—you may consider yourself an ultra-efficient person, a master multitasker. But regardless of how "in control" you feel in the moment, your split focus may actually be a hindrance, not a help. "Multitasking doesn't work, even if it feels like it's working," says Marc Berman, PhD, a cognitive neuroscientist at the University of Michigan who has researched the mind's ability to shift focus.

While it often feels like you're able to effectively juggle many tasks, most of us are unable to seamlessly do a few things at once: when you're not giving your full attention to any one thing, chances are nothing gets done quite as well, or with the care that it should. In fact, a recent study found that just 5 percent of the population is what researchers refer to as "super-taskers," people who can successfully engage in multiple activities at once. What does this mean for the rest of us? That it's best to focus on one thing at a time.

282 Grow your compassion by giving others your attention

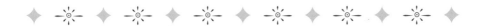

YOU DON'T THINK TWICE ABOUT running to your best friend's side when she has a problem, and you've got a generous supply of compassion for the other important people in your life. But what about everyone else? Does your kindness reach all of the people you meet? If your compassion isn't universal, there's one simple way to extend this warmth to everyone you encounter: simply give them your undivided attention, says Sharon Salzberg, author of *Real Happiness: Learning the Power of Meditation.*

According to Salzberg, there are a lot of people who we feel don't "matter" to us as much as others do. If you've already made this decision about them—that you don't like or respect or care about them—then when you're around them, you're not being present in your own life or treating those around you with respect, kindness, and understanding.

The next time you catch yourself doing this, turn it around. For example, Salzberg says, "if somebody is talking to me and I find myself not paying attention, hoping that they'll hurry up, then I try to really center and pay attention to them. If I pay more attention to that person, I'm able to see what state they're in and actually hear what they're saying." By giving everyone your full attention, you'll gain a bit more patience and compassion by making another person feel heard.

283 De-escalate your workouts for unexpected results

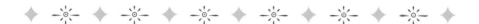

IF YOUR GOAL IS TO DROP pounds, then you probably want to stick with the exercise philosophy of working out harder and faster for best results. But if you're looking for other fitness benefits, like an immunity boost, a reduction in pain, or a decrease in stress levels, slow movements—like yoga and Tai Chi—may be best. According to Alan Fogel, PhD, professor of psychology at The University of Utah and author of *The Psychophysiology of Self-Awareness: Rediscovering the Lost Art of Body Sense,* a greater mind-body connection is what sets these slow movements apart from other types of exercise.

The mind-body link is formed when you must pay close attention to how your body moves and where it is in space. As you test yourself to move with a slow flow, to balance, and to feel subtle shifts in your placement, you actually strengthen your brain's neuro-network, says Fogel. This soft focus on slow movement leads to a greater awareness and a number of health benefits, including fewer colds and less stress. Says Fogel, "There are positive effects of paying attention to how you're moving. By slowing down, you're able to come back to yourself."

284 Stop stress with a new hobby

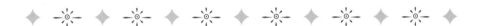

IF YOU THINK THAT THERE'S NO room in your life for a hobby, it's a clear indication that you need to make some calendar space. Pastimes like playing guitar, making crafts, and gardening provide a healthy and fun distraction from your daily grind. But even more importantly, hobbies help you relax, says Gabriela Corá, MD, MBA, founder of the Executive Health & Wealth Institute in Miami, Florida, and author of *Leading Under Pressure.*

"A hobby doesn't put any pressure on you—it's just something that you find enjoyable and interesting," explains Corá. That's why a sport or other activity that leaves you feeling competitive—even with yourself—may not be the best diversion if you're seeking an escape. In order to unwind, your hobby should give you pleasure in the process, regardless of outcome. "Find an activity that fully captures your attention, so that you lose track of everything else that's going on," suggests Corá, who believes that repetitive tasks, like knitting, can impart an even greater sense of calm than other pastimes. As you immerse yourself in your hobby, you may be too preoccupied to realize that your worries and stress are melting away.

285 Protect your mind one drink at a time

ENJOYING A GLASS OF WINE
with dinner—or two glasses if you're male—
can benefit your heart health, and new
studies show that this moderate amount of
alcohol consumption is good for your brain,
too. According to a large-scale study from
Norway, which tracked the drinking habits
and health of more than 5,000 people for
seven years, scientists found that those who
drank in moderation, particularly women,
experienced fewer declines in cognitive
function. This backs up other research that
has found that moderate drinking protects
the brain from such conditions as dementia
and Alzheimer's disease and also leads to
improvements in overall cognitive function.
A drink or so a day brings on the best health
effects compared to drinking heavily or not
at all.

286 Calmness is just a breath away

EXERCISE IS NOT ONLY EXCELLENT for increasing physical fitness; it's also good for your mind. By pushing your physical limits, you build mental strength and resilience, too, says Bryan Kest, creator of Power Yoga.

For instance, if you place your body in challenging positions in a yoga class, says Kest, you can learn to better handle your response to stress. During a class, Kest reminds students to check in with their mind and breath. "If your breath gets erratic and choppy, it may mean that you're scared; if you're angry, it can become fast. When you're calm and peaceful, so is your breath," says Kest. Focusing on and regulating your breath can also help you maintain your composure in difficult situations in your day-to-day life, be it a tough conversation with your boss or a frustrating commute.

287

Treat allergies to ease depression

ALLERGIES GOT YOU DOWN?

According to researchers at the University of Maryland School of Medicine, sniffles and sneezing may be the least of your problems if you have allergies brought on by ragweed or tree pollen. In a recent study, researchers found that untreated allergies to these plants may increase incidence of depression, particularly when pollen counts are at their peak. In fact, in a trial that recruited people who were depressed or suffering from bipolar disorder, more than half of the people had these allergies, and their depression rates increased with allergy season. The research team is still trying to find hard evidence to show that simply treating allergies is enough to improve mood, but that's what they expect to find. If your allergies start to flare up, reach for a tissue, as well as an anti-allergen, such as Claritin.

288 Don't sabotage your workout results

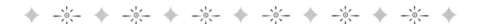

IF YOU'RE CURRENTLY WORKING out, congratulations and keep it up! Just don't use your exercise regimen as an excuse to limit other daily activity. For instance, if you go for a run each morning, you may be tempted to drive on errands you used to walk—because, after all, you've done your exercise for the day. But dropping daily activities means you'll cancel out the calories burned during exercise. If you start moving less, you may not lose the weight you want, and, in some cases, you may even gain more.

In a recent U.K. study, co-authored by Eirini Manthou, a researcher in exercise and nutrition at the University of Glasgow, Scotland, thirty-four overweight women completed the same 150-minute-a-week exercise program. All worked out regularly, but some women lost up to seven pounds of body fat, while others gained up to five. Manthou's take on the results: the women who lost the most were the ones who maintained or increased their physical activity outside of the gym; the women who gained weight had cut back on their activity levels outside of the gym.

To increase your daily activity, simply look for opportunities to walk, stand, and take the stairs more. Put reminders in your calendar during the workday to stand up and take a lap around the office. Commit to walking to the store instead of driving. Or add an extra hour of housework (cleaning, decluttering, etc.) each week. Whether you work out or not, simply getting out of your chair more frequently can refresh your mind and help you burn more calories.

289 Reach out and touch someone

RESEARCH SHOWS THAT THE
power of touch is so great, it can stimulate
the brain to reduce stress hormones, release
a bonding chemical, and ease feelings of
depression. And large gestures aren't the only
ones that make a difference, says Matthew
Hertenstein, PhD, head of DePauw University's Touch and Emotion Lab. Even fleeting
touches, like a pat on the back or a touch on
the elbow, can invoke a deep reaction.

Yet, as a culture, we're touching one another
less and less. In fact, says Hertenstein, many
people without romantic partners experience no touch throughout the day, which
means missing out on a major source of
positive emotions. The reasons for this shift
to a low-contact society are plenty. But there
are lots of appropriate places for touch: you
can hug friends, squeeze your child's arm
in encouragement, or offer your jogging
partner a high five after a long run.

290 Embrace your imper- fections

YOU MAY STRIVE TO BE THE BEST at everything you do. But if you're intent on being perfect all of the time, you may be missing out on leading a truly authentic life, one in which you're defined by the traits you consider good *and* the ones you sometimes wish you didn't have. "To find your 'true self,' you've got to get used to the fact that you are less than perfect. That's what it means to be human," says Parker Palmer, PhD, author of *A Hidden Wholeness: The Journey Toward an Undivided Life* and founder of the Center for Courage and Renewal, an organization devoted to helping people to bring positive change to their lives. In order to act and think as your own independent self, you must accept that imperfection is okay—it's simply part of the human condition. That doesn't mean that trying to correct bad habits or aim higher with your goals is a negative thing, but by accepting your quirks and limitations, you'll be less hard on yourself and more true to the person you really are.

291 Gain new perspective with creativity

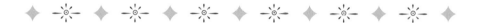

THERE'S A HIDDEN BENEFIT TO pursuing creative pastimes, like taking a dance workshop or setting aside an evening each week to draw or write. When your creativity flows, your mind slows down and your senses open up. According to Rikki Asher, EdD, director of art education at Queens College and an occasional presenter at the Omega Institute for Holistic Studies, creative time also encourages more thoughtful responses to the environment, other people, and even yourself.

To explain this change in mentality, which is a lot like meditation, Asher draws on an image used by one of her teachers, which likens the mind to a glass of muddy water: when it's constantly stirred, the water remains foggy; but when it's left alone, the liquid and dirt separate, and the water becomes clearer. "Like the mud, our thoughts begin to settle when we sit for a few minutes," says Asher. To experience this shift, pull out a drawing pad or put on music you like to dance to, then allow yourself to get caught up in the activity. Your thoughts may fade as you work, but when you come back to them, you'll see them with a fresh perspective.

292 Gossiping can be good

CHANCES ARE YOU'VE PROBABLY been told that it's not nice to talk about other people. But with the right attitude, conversing about others is actually a good thing. That's because there's a difference between praising people who aren't present and gossiping about their foibles behind their backs. While the latter can breed negativity for all, talking about a person in a positive way can boost your mood, say researchers from Staffordshire University. In one study, people were asked to talk about a fictional person in either a negative or positive way. Afterward, although the person being gossiped about was imaginary, the people who had had more upbeat conversations experienced a boost in self-esteem. Overall, gossipers report feeling a higher degree of social support than less chatty types, but when you start talking about someone else, be sure the conversation is one you'd be happy with that person overhearing.

293 Breathe your way to better perspective

IF YOU'VE EVER TAKEN A YOGA class, you know that breath plays a central role in the practice. In fact, many eastern traditions—including meditation and Tai Chi—have a strong emphasis on breath. The act of deeply inhaling and exhaling can slow the pulse and relax the body, but it also has significant mental effects, says Ayurvedic medicine teacher Laura Plumb, cofounder of the Deep Yoga School of Healing Arts in San Diego. Observing your breath helps you to turn your focus inward and give you perspective, says Plumb. The air is able to sustain you, although it comes and goes. Spending a few minutes of each day observing this phenomenon can be especially useful when you're confused or doubtful and need help trying to find your "true self."

294 Get a great-smelling home, sans chemicals

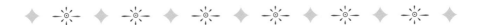

YOU KNOW THAT MAGIC ODOR- eliminator you use to mask stale smells when you don't have time to clean the house? Turns out that breathing in those aromatic sprays, powders, and plug-ins has been linked to several health hazards, from allergies to cancer. To avoid these toxins and get a fresh-smelling home, take a page from generations past, says Cassidy Randall, program and outreach coordinator for Women's Voices for the Earth, a watchdog organization for the environment.

For instance, sprinkle baking soda or coffee grounds in a smelly garbage can, both of which are effective at tempering trash bin odors. You can also ameliorate a pungent garbage disposal by dropping a lemon wedge down the drain, and deodorize a carpet by sprinkling it with baking soda, then vacuuming it a few hours later. To give your home an all-over enticing aroma, buy fresh flowers or bake spices in the oven, says Randall. Finally, when doing laundry, skip the fabric softener and add ½ cup white distilled vinegar to the rinse cycle of your washer, then let your clothing dry outside—you can skip the dryer sheet and your fabrics will pick up the clean scent of the outdoors.

295 Close friends affect health and happiness

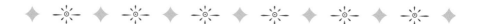

RESEARCH HAS SHOWN THAT our social networks influence everything, from how healthy we are to whether or not we vote in an election. But with sites like Facebook allowing us to keep in touch with more people than ever before, how does our expanding circle of "friends" affect us? Not as much as you might think, it turns out. "Facebook friends don't have the same influence as friends you spend time with in person," says James Fowler, PhD, professor at the University of California, San Diego, and co-author of *Connected: The Surprising Power of Our Social Networks and How They Shape Our Lives.*

When Fowler examined friend networks on sites like Facebook, he found that the influences he often saw in real-life networks didn't exist between a person and all of his or her contacts. But, when he scaled down the size of a network to just those people who were tagged in one another's photos, the real-life models of social influence applied. So, even if your online friends have habits you don't want to rub off on you or opinions you think are off-base, chances are that you will remain unaffected. Only the friends we spend time with more directly affect our health and happiness.

296 Home-cooked meals are best

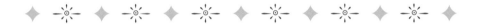

DON'T LET A BUSY SCHEDULE keep you from cooking. "It's fine to take shortcuts," says Bonnie Taub-Dix, MA, RD, CDN, a practicing dietician with more than thirty-five years of experience and author of *Read It Before You Eat It*. It takes just a few minutes to whip up a healthy, nutritious meal that tastes great and costs a fraction of what you'd pay for take-out.

Although fresh produce is best, when you're in a time crunch, frozen fruits and veggies are fine, says Taub-Dix. Canned foods are alright, too, so long as they don't have too many additives, like extra salt or sugar—most offer a substantial helping of nutrients and vitamins without the labor of chopping or sautéing. And, buying a prepared main course—like a roasted chicken—will allow you more time to focus on preparing fresh side dishes, like grilled asparagus or a large salad.

Planning ahead also makes it easier to pull together quick meals. "When you have extra time, buy twice as many vegetables as you need and cut them all up at once," suggests Taub-Dix. This way, they'll be chopped for the week; if you don't use them quickly enough, you can always freeze the veggies—they'll be ready to eat as soon as you thaw them. Another handy tip: make more than you need so you'll have leftovers for tomorrow!

297 Sleep better, feel better

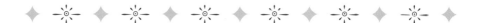

IT'S EASY TO TAKE SLEEP FOR granted, so long as you're getting enough Zs. But if you have trouble falling asleep, suffer through restless nights, or wake too early, you start to appreciate just how important sleep is for resetting your body and mind, giving you energy, and keeping your immune system functioning. If you're having trouble sleeping, your evening habits may be a part of the problem, says Mark Liponis, MD, author of *UltraLongevity*. You can take some simple steps to get a better night's sleep.

Create a sleeping space that is cool, dark, and quiet, says Liponis. Getting too warm while you sleep is one reason many people wake during the night or have a restless slumber, and light and sound can be equally disruptive. Then, pay attention to your body's natural rhythms: if you get drowsy at 10:30 P.M., don't force yourself to stay up until midnight. Doing so will only make you feel sleep-deprived. If your partner snores or is a restless sleeper, see if you can make adjustments that help him or her—and you—have a more restful night.

298 Beat high blood pressure by eating beets

NEXT TIME YOU'RE AT A JUICE bar, ask for a beverage with beet juice in it: the deep-red root vegetable will add sweetness to your drink and help manage your blood pressure. In fact, researchers at the William Harvey Research Institute in London found that just 250 milliliters of beetroot juice, or a little more than a cup, is as effective at lowering blood pressure as one commonly prescribed medication. According to the National Institutes of Health, one in four Americans suffers from hypertension—a serious condition that can increase your risk of heart disease or stroke—so if your doctor wants to discuss treatment options, consider this natural approach.

299 Do a good deed, get a good workout

IF YOU WANT TO INCREASE YOUR endurance, try harnessing the connection between your mind and body. Researchers at Harvard University recently found that exercisers who did a good deed—or even imagined themselves doing one—had a boost in physical endurance.

In the study, people were given a dollar and the choice to either keep it or donate it to charity, then they were asked to hold a hand weight for as long as they could. The ones who donated the money were able to hold on longer, indicating that generosity can lead to improved willpower and an ability to put up with discomfort for longer. In psychological terms, this boost is called moral transformation—the idea is that by doing good deeds and helping others you feel better about your abilities, resulting in increased confidence, willpower, and stamina for other tasks.

300 Grow older, wiser, and happier

THE SAYING GOES, "OLDER AND wiser." But, according to new research, you can add happier to the list, too. Based on the work of Ulrich Orth, PhD, a research professor in the University of Basel's department of psychology, self-esteem tends to increase with age until around sixty, and there are ways to keep your spirits high for even longer.

Independence is one way to boost happiness as you grow older—in the study, people who were healthy and wealthy enough to do as they pleased had higher self-esteem than those who didn't. But simply growing your support system can boost esteem, according to other research. If you focus on building a sense of community as you age, such as becoming involved in a church group or mentoring organization, or continuing to plan regular outings with friends, you, too, can age with grace and joy.

301 Train your brain to stay calm

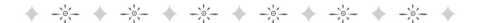

SOMETIMES, THINGS THAT SEEM like they should be relaxing aren't. Just think about that last massage you got, when your mind was racing the whole time. But it doesn't take much to get in the Zen zone, according to Linda Lantieri, director of The Inner Resilience Program, an organization focused on building emotional strength in school teachers. Chances are that you can easily identify a few activities that inspire what Lantieri calls "relaxed alertness," the state of being fully aware and awake, but not at all stressed. Listening to music, taking a nature walk, or praying may inspire this state—whatever it is, the more often you do the activity, the better the effects on the rest of your life.

"These activities are good in and of themselves, but because the brain is strengthened by experience, the idea is that over time, you'll be able to call on this relaxed state even when you're in a more stressful situation," says Lantieri. "By adding real relaxation to your day, you're not just changing habits—you're actually changing the structure of your brain."

For best results, find daily ways to enter this worry-free state. Meditation might work well for you, or you might need a more active hobby, like scrapbooking, to strengthen your sense of calm. Over time, the relaxing response will become second nature, says Lantieri. You'll not only be less reactive to daily stressors, but also be better prepared to handle bigger challenges.

302 De-stress to cure PMS

YOU'RE CRANKY, TIRED, AND dreaming about chocolate. If you're female (or are with a woman who is demonstrating all of these symptoms), you know this could only mean one thing—it's that time of the month. Although doctors estimate that between 40 and 60 percent of reproductive age women suffer from PMS, with symptoms ranging from mood swings to cravings, little is known about the actual causes of the condition or how to treat it. However, one recent study from the Eunice Kennedy Shriver National Institute of Child Health and Human Development has found one thing that definitely makes PMS worse: stress.

In the study, 259 women were asked about their stress levels at different times of their cycle. The women who reported the highest levels of perceived stress also reported the most menstrual symptoms, and the severest. Researchers believe that stress reduction programs may help PMS, so try engaging in sports or other hobbies to get some relief.

303 The benefits of black rice

YOU MADE THE SWITCH FROM
white rice a few years back when nutritionists found that the brown variety contained
higher levels of antioxidants, which are
important for counteracting free radicals in
the body, such as those that cause cancer. Now, it may be time to switch to yet
another color of the grain: black. Recent
research from scientists at Louisiana State
University's food sciences department shows
that black rice has more antioxidants than
brown rice, and it even beats out the superfood blueberries. Black rice has a stronger
flavor than either brown or white rice, but
it can be used in combination with brown
rice to neutralize the taste. The grain has
long been available at specialty stores, but
you can now find it in the aisles of more
and more traditional supermarkets, too.

304 Go from skinny-fat to skinny-strong

HERE'S ANOTHER REASON TO pump iron: research shows that dieting alone isn't enough to keep type 2 diabetes at bay. In a study of more than 14,500 people, scientists found that both thin and overweight people with below average muscle tone had insulin resistance, a precursor to type 2 diabetes. And, according to a recent Mayo Clinic study of more than six thousand non-obese adults, thin people who have a high percentage of body fat were more at risk for heart problems, too. To boost your muscle tone quickly, aim for two to three sessions of full-body strength training each week. You can choose between weight lifting, resistance bands, kettlebells, bootcamp-style workouts, and even Pilates and yoga to both reduce your risk of illness and get a toned physique.

305 Be scent-savvy to have sweeter dreams

IF YOU'VE HAD A SLEW OF BAD dreams, you may want to move your dirty clothes hamper or trash can a bit farther away from your bed: German researchers have found that just as pleasant aromas and smelly odors influence your mood while you're awake, these fragrances can produce the same sort of effects while you sleep. This means that your dreams are colored by the air you breathe. In the German study, people who were exposed to a scent while they slept—either roses or rotten eggs—reported having dreams that were either positive or negative, with the scents matching the moods you'd expect. Even if a bad scent isn't to blame for your restless nights, place a fragrant bouquet in your room. The scent may influence your dreams, and studies show that simply seeing flowers—such as before you fall asleep or once you wake—can improve your mood.

306 Don't dwell on goofs and gaffes

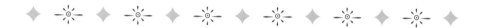

WE'VE ALL DONE IT. WE'VE ALL tripped on a stair, fumbled our words, or committed some other momentarily mortifying blunder. The trick to a quick recovery is learning not to be too hard on yourself. Whoever witnessed your faux pas probably didn't pay it much mind. In fact, as you're replaying the event in your head, chances are everyone else has already moved on— if their attention lingered at all.

"If you make a misstep, it's likely others have experienced those same certain disasters," says Thomas D. Gilovich, PhD, professor and chair of the Cornell University psychology department. "Because of that, they're usually much more empathic than you might anticipate."

Not convinced? Just try to recall the last time you saw someone commit an embarrassing error. It's probably not that easy, and even if you can remember a friend spilling a glass of wine, or a stranger slipping on a patch of ice, chances are you were more sympathetic than scornful.

Also, keep in mind that what we find embarrassing may not even register with others. "If you have a bad hair day and feel like you can't go out, it's likely that other people won't even notice that you look different than on any other day," says Gilovich.

Honest mistakes are just a part of life. "Take it with a grain of salt," recommends Gilovich. "If there's something to learn from it, put it in the file. If not, move on."

307 Add sleep to your weight-loss plan

IF YOU WANT TO LOSE WEIGHT, make sure you're getting your Zs. According-ing to a recent study from France, sleep-deprived people eat more than well-rested ones. Scientists have long known that poor sleep habits can increase the risk of becoming overweight, but in this study, researchers found that people who were limited to four hours of sleep per night consumed almost six hundred calories more the next day than they did follow-ing a full night's sleep. They also reported being hungrier throughout the day. All of the extra food the short sleepers took in did help fuel a small increase in activity, but only enough to burn off fifty of those extra calories. To be sure you're setting yourself up for healthy weight success, aim for around seven hours of sleep each night.

308 Take a break from your PDA

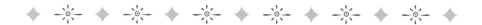

"BLACKBERRYITIS," COMMONLY defined as an unnatural obsession with one's PDA, has been known to cause dinner table disputes and sleepless nights. But that constant typing and scrolling can bring on physical symptoms, too, most commonly pain in the thumbs, hands, and neck. "These handheld devices should be used as a complement to work on a computer, not an alternative," says Karen Jacobs, EdD, OTR/L a clinical professor of occupational therapy at Boston University. If you suffer from any of the above, it may be time to rethink how you use your smartphone or hand-held organizer.

"To cut down on your PDA use, use the device to quickly check your messages, but not to send them," suggests Jacobs. "Send most of your e-mails from a regular computer, which is designed for longer periods of use." If you use your handheld gadget to jot down notes, give your fingers a break by using the voice-memo function found on most phones and digital assistants—simply speak your message and retrieve it later. When you must type, use your index fingers in addition to your thumbs, says Jacobs, and take frequent breaks. Finally, hold the device high and close enough that you can see the screen without scrunching your neck.

309 Free yourself from the fear of failure

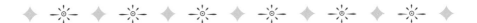

YOU SKIPPED A RECENT SKI TRIP because you were too embarrassed to fall in front of your friends; you were so worried about burning a cake that you . . . burned the cake. If these scenarios sound familiar, you may suffer from a fear of failure. "Fear of failure is related to a form of perfectionism, specifically what researchers refer to as socially prescribed perfectionism," says David E. Conroy, PhD, associate professor of kinesiology and human development and family studies at The Pennsylvania State University. Fear of failure can prevent you from trying new things, or psyche you out so much that you really do make mistakes.

According to Conroy, fear of failure takes root in early childhood as children develop a sense of self, internalize standards for their behavior, and find ways to evaluate how well they meet those goals. Conroy has found that young athletes who felt their coaches were critical and blaming on the field became more critical of themselves.

To minimize fear of failure, don't blow mistakes or errors out of proportion, and be realistic about your expectations. Taking a few spills on the bunny slope is a natural part of learning to ski, and a well-done cake is better than no cake at all! If you're still feeling uncertain, put yourself in someone else's shoes—chances are you wouldn't judge a person harshly for trying to learn something new or fumbling every once in a while. Take it easy on yourself.

310

Make one small change to wake rested

YOU'RE TIRED EACH MORNING, even though you're going to bed at a reasonable time and getting in the recommended seven or more hours of sleep. What gives? One of the most common sleep disruptors is the mid-slumber bathroom break, says Mark Liponis, MD, corporate medical director of Canyon Ranch health resorts and author of *UltraLongevity*. According to Liponis, getting up isn't the problem—but turning on a light to illuminate your trip is. Bright light affects the body's clock—the pineal gland, in the brain. When light is detected, your body shuts off production of melatonin, the sleep hormone, making it hard to fall back asleep. To avoid this problem, install dim blue-tinted night-lights along your path to the bathroom. Also, limit fluids after 8 P.M. to limit your need to get up at all.

311

To speed up weight loss, spice up your food

IF YOU LOVE TO DOUSE YOUR food in Tabasco sauce, you're in luck—that spicy flavor does a whole lot more than just bring a flush to your face: according to several studies, capsaicin, the active ingredient in chili peppers, actually helps speed up weight loss. When you eat a spicy pepper—and in particular the white membrane that holds the seeds in place inside the plant, which has the highest levels of capsaicin—your metabolism increases, you burn more calories, and you oxidize more fat. And, in a recent study, capsaicin actually reduced appetite, too, causing people to eat less. If you get too much spice in a bite, drink cold milk. Researchers have found it more effective than water at putting out the fire in your mouth.

312

Quick tips for a clear complexion

FEW PEOPLE ARE BORN WITH perfect skin, but with a bit of effort, anyone can have a clear complexion, says Sonia Badreshia-Bansal, MD, a dermatologist who teaches at the University of California, San Francisco. According to Badreshia-Bansal, a diet high in antioxidants—think lots of fruits and veggies—can help regulate insulin levels and deter breakouts. Alternately, fried foods or foods high in fat or sugar provoke more fluctuations in insulin levels, which can cause your skin to suffer.

If you do have a breakout, avoid over-scrubbing, over-exfoliating, or otherwise irritating your skin, which can lead to more sensitivity and breakouts. Instead, says Badreshia-Bansal, treat problematic pimples with a benzoyl peroxide–based spot treatment—simply dab a small dot of the drying cream on the blemish until it disappears, which will take about two or three days.

313 Eat nuts for a healthy heart

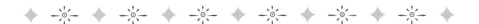

IF YOU HAVE A FAMILY HISTORY of heart disease, consider switching to a diet low in saturated fat, cholesterol, and sodium to lower the amount of fat found in the blood and to moderate cholesterol levels. This heart-healthy diet may sound somewhat limiting, but this type of meal plan isn't only about cutting out pleasurable foods. There are several delicious, healthy foods you can add for great benefits. For example, many types of nuts can actually aid in lowering fat levels, says Joan Sabaté, MD, DrPH, chair and professor of nutrition at Loma Linda University's School of Public Health.

Recently, Sabaté compiled the results of twenty-five nut consumption trials and found that although nuts contain a relatively high amount of fat, eating certain varieties led to a marked improvement in blood lipid levels and a decrease in cholesterol. To naturally lower your risk of heart disease, reach for a handful of almonds, walnuts, peanuts, pecans, or pistachios. Sabaté recommends eating 1 ½ to 2 ½ ounces a day, or about ⅓ to ½ cup. For best health results, choose nuts that are raw or dry roasted.

314 Find clarity by changing your routine

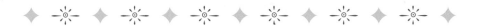

YOU'VE PROBABLY BEEN TOLD to "step away from the situation" when you need to make a big decision. Turns out, this advice is spot on, and works best if you interpret it literally: according to Sarah Livia Szekely Brightwood, who runs Rancho la Puerta, a fitness spa and retreat in Mexico, at critical moments in your life, changing your environment can give you the space you need to make a decision. "Being away from everyday routines allows you to shift your perspective—you're better able to identify your place in the grand scheme of things, to see from the outside where you fit."

Even an afternoon or weekend off from your daily routine can help bring you clarity, says Brightwood, but for major transitions, a full week is best. She's found that it takes about three days to shed your worries and come back to a centered place. If heading off to a full-service retreat isn't possible, try a DIY escape: plan a weekend away with your favorite friends, making sure to incorporate learning opportunities, such as taking an art class or trying kayaking for the first time. As you feel supported, challenged, and inspired, you'll be able to access your inner thoughts on the decision at hand and renew your inner strength.

315

Achieve domestic bliss with division of labor

IF YOU'RE AT YOUR WIT'S END trying to get your significant other to pick up his or her socks, team up and do it together: According to a recent study from Canada, couples who join forces to keep the house clean report higher levels of happiness in their relationships. In the report, which surveyed thousands of people, when just one partner was responsible for the housework, couples were more stressed and less satisfied with life. They measured a variety of scenarios—with both people working or just one, and with one or both cleaning—and found the highest levels of contentment and lowest levels of stress among households where chores were split between two partners. If your home life could benefit from more happiness, split up the cleaning, cooking, and childcare responsibilities.

316

Eat familiar foods to shed pounds

YOU MAY BE TEMPTED TO TRY any new snacks you see in the low-calorie aisle of your grocery store, but if you're trying to lose weight, it's best to limit the number of new foods you add to your diet. In his research, Jeff Brunstrom, PhD, a behavioral nutrition researcher at the University of Bristol, has found that people often underestimate how satisfying a new food may be, causing them to eat more than they need. If you're getting bored with your diet, swapping a few items at a time is okay, but test small portions to learn the best amount to eat. Most importantly, don't overhaul your whole diet, or you may wind up eating even more calories than you were before.

317 Why you should drink decaf

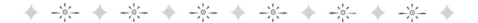

DON'T LISTEN TO THE NAYSAYERS telling you that coffee is bad for you. Java naturally contains polyphenols, compounds that actually *boost* health, says Peter Rogers, PhD, head of the department of experimental psychology at the University of Bristol. Caffeine content, it turns out, is the real culprit behind coffee's bad rap.

Caffeine may give you extra pep, but it comes at a price: For starters, a recent study co-authored by Rogers shows that the feeling of alertness people get may actually be due to low levels of anxiety brought on by caffeine. Also, caffeine raises blood pressure,

says Rogers. While polyphenols appear to mitigate the negative effects of high blood pressure, lessening your risk of cardiovascular disease or early cognitive decline, you should still try to avoid hypertension in the first place.

Finally, caffeine really can become an addiction, as you know all too well if you've ever endured a throbbing headache after missing your morning cup. If you don't want to give up your morning ritual—and want the health benefits of coffee—try switching to decaf and using exercise and adequate sleep as a natural source of energy.

318 Lift sadness with rose oil

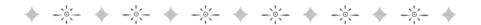

SCENT HAS THE UNIQUE ABILITY to transport you to another time and place. For example, a whiff of a particular sunblock may send you back to a summer spent at the shore. It's no surprise then that rose essential oil is recommended for times of emotional stress. The sweet smell of the oil—which may remind you of tender occasions—calms the psyche, says Hope Gillerman, a holistic healer and creator of a line of essential oil–based remedies and care products.

Rose is one of the more expensive essential oils—it takes barrels of petals to produce a small vial of oil—but in times of grief, such as when coping with loss or heartache, it's a very effective way to soothe the soul. "It's like an essential oil hug," says Gillerman.

For a daily dose, mix a half teaspoon of rose oil with a small bottle of unscented body oil and rub the blend on your chest and shoulders, where it will be absorbed by the skin and also primed for inhalation. Or, create a perfume-like spray that you can carry with you made of one part rose, three parts jojoba oil. (Oil and water, of course, don't mix, so you need an oil or oil-based lotion to dilute an essential oil.) When you start to feel sad, spritz the scent and breathe it in. If cost is prohibitive, try geranium or orange essential oils, both of which are less expensive but still have antidepressant properties.

319 Laugh more to live longer

IF YOU'RE LOOKING TO PRESERVE your health, you might try a new diet or exercise plan, both of which have been proven to add years to your life. But longevity could be just a joke away, as science now shows that laughter can significantly improve overall health. Researchers in Norway recently found that a sense of humor appears to buffer your body from stress-related conditions, like heart disease and high blood pressure. In the study, scientists reported that keeping a sense of humor appeared to improve terminal patients' rate of survival by 31 percent. To make major gains in your longevity, lighten up—by finding more things to laugh about in everyday life, you'll actually be improving your health.

320 Eat small meals to stay slim *and* healthy

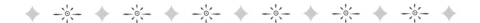

OVEREATING NOT ONLY LEAVES you with a bellyache, it also puts you more at risk of developing serious health problems. In addition to packing on unwanted pounds—and being overweight or obese comes with its own set of health concerns—the very act of overeating can cause your immune system to turn on you, no matter what your size or shape.

"A big meal is stressful on the body and it triggers the immune system to over-react," says Mark Liponis, MD, author of *UltraLongevity*. "This overreaction causes inflammation, and inflammation is the central feature of all diseases that affect us in mid-life and beyond, such as heart disease and diabetes."

To reduce inflammation, eat small meals throughout the day, rather than a couple of large ones. Liponis suggests adopting a "grazing strategy," eating several small portions every couple of hours. If you'd rather have a true breakfast, lunch, and dinner, then snack on healthy foods between meals—doing so may help you to eat less at mealtimes, and ultimately stay healthier and slimmer.

321

Get two-for-one workout results

IF YOU DON'T HAVE TIME TO FIT in separate cardio and resistance training sessions, double up. According to Michele Olson, PhD, professor of exercise science at the Auburn University at Montgomery, combining strength training with aerobic activity helps you to maximize your time without taking away from your target strength gains or calorie burn.

If you have a handful of resistance moves you like, start your workout with those, suggests Olson. You'll build strength and warm up your muscles for an intense cardio workout. Or, boost your heart rate during resistance training: lift faster than usual, add cardio drills (like jumping jacks) between sets, or try a cardiovascular resistance workout, like moves done with kettlebells. No matter how you combine the two, shoot for the American College of Sports Medicine's recommended 150 minutes or more of fitness a week.

322 Whole foods keep you healthy

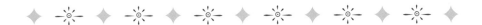

WHAT SHOULD YOU CONSUME to ward off a cold? A tall glass of OJ might be the first thing that comes to mind, thanks to its high vitamin C content. But you'd be better off eating the entire orange, says Gregory G. Freund, MD, head of pathology at the University of Illinois at Urbana-Champaign's College of Medicine. The white part of an orange peel and other fruit skins—parts that are commonly discarded when a fruit is turned into juice—are rich in pectin, a type of soluble fiber. In his work, Freund has linked soluble fiber with improved immunity—the more you eat, the less susceptible you'll be to illness.

Increasing your fiber intake sounds easy enough. But fiber comes in both soluble and insoluble forms, and only the soluble sort has been linked to improved immunity. "Soluble means it likes to be in a wetter environment," says Freund, like fruits, vegetables, and beans. So, while insoluble fiber—such as that found in high-fiber foods like packaged cereals—helps with digestion and other aspects of health, it won't necessarily boost immunity.

Citrus fruits, apples, and strawberries contain high levels of soluble fiber, and so do vegetables like broccoli, peas, potatoes, and carrots. And, these foods all contain other nutrients that have been linked to immunity, such as vitamins A, C, and E, to name a few. Many packaged foods do not separate fiber content by soluble and insoluble fiber, so if in doubt, consult a nutrition guide.

323

Sigh your way to stronger lungs

IF YOU GET SIDE STITCHES WHEN you work out, your breathing muscles may not be as in shape as the rest of your body. Exercise can help to train the respiratory muscles over time, but you can also increase breath control without working up a sweat, says Thomas Vanhecke, MD, a cardiologist at William Beaumont Hospital in Royal Oak, Michigan.

"Although sighs are often regarded as a sign of boredom or tiredness, they also offer a significant benefit for respiratory mechanics," says Vanhecke. A sigh is defined as a breath three times larger than a normal breath. You probably already sigh ten to twelve times an hour, but increasing this amount may help strengthen your breath. If you'd rather have an official routine, follow a guided meditation that emphasizes sigh-like deep breathing. Or, simply focus on taking long and controlled inhales and exhales. Start by breathing in for a count of four and out for a count of four, moving up to six, then eight, and so on.

324 Remember to laugh—not just cry—with your friends

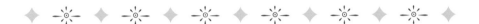

TURNING TO A FRIEND FOR support can bring you closer when you've hit a rough patch in life—after all, that's what friends are for. But rehashing the details of a negative experience will leave you both feeling down in the long run. Amanda Rose, PhD, associate professor in the University of Missouri's department of psychological sciences, has studied the effects of co-rumination, where two or more people analyze and dwell on a specific problem. In her studies, she found that people who spend a lot of time doing this had strong relationships but, interestingly, they also had higher levels of stress.

How can you keep a healthy balance? "For friendships to be close and intimate, it's important to share sad feelings when they come up," says Rose, just don't go overboard. "Doing so in moderation allows feelings of closeness in friendship but alleviates the downsides—such as depression and anxiety—associated with co-ruminating," she says.

According to Rose, positive feelings in the friendship likely stem from talking and sharing. To feel inspired, rather than defeated, steer talk toward your hopes and dreams or other positive topics. You'll continue to feel connected to your friend, but the effects of the conversation on your mood—and hers—will be more pleasant.

325 Cranberries can benefit health year-round

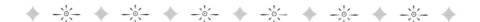

WHOLE CRANBERRIES ARE OFTEN available only in the fall, around Thanksgiving and the holidays, when the berries are ripe and cranberry sauce is a staple on most tables. But cranberries are a smart option year-round. They pack a health punch powerful enough to rival the most popular superfoods. Serving to serving, cranberries contain more phenols—a type of antioxidant—than blueberries, apples, red grapes, and strawberries, according to Diane L. McKay, PhD, a scientist at Tufts University's Antioxidants Research Laboratory who has studied the fruit.

Luckily, the health benefits found in cranberries are still present in the juice and dried fruit, and because whole cranberries are quite tart, these alternatives may actually be more palatable. "Specific cranberry products like dried, sweetened cranberries and cranberry juice cocktail have been recognized by the American Heart Association as 'heart healthy' based on their nutrient composition," says McKay, and cranberries and cranberry products may help lower blood pressure and reduce artery hardening. Cranberries and their derivatives are also associated with the prevention of urinary tract infections and stomach ulcers, as well as improved oral hygiene. And, dried cranberries provide more than 10 percent of the recommended dietary allowance of fiber and cranberry juice cocktail contains more than 100 percent of the recommended dietary allowance of vitamin C.

Look for the juices and dried fruits with the least amount of added sugar. A standard rule is that most adults should consume the equivalent of about 2 cups of fruit daily: in general, 1 cup of 100 percent fruit juice, or ½ cup of dried fruit can be considered 1 cup from the fruit group.

326 Take it easy to prevent chronic pain

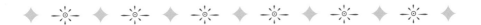

CHRONIC PAIN IS TOUGH TO treat, but it's often possible to prevent. According to Paul L. Durham, PhD, director of the Center for Biomedical and Life Sciences at Missouri State University, you can keep an acute injury—like a sore tooth or achy knee—from turning into a more chronic condition simply by getting enough rest.

"When you don't let your body restore itself, it can't heal," says Durham. Rejuvenation can come in two different ways: through actual sleep, or just from taking it easy. For example, if you hit your tooth, you'll have inflammation and pain to help remind you not to use it for the first twenty-four hours or so, says Durham. But if you ignore your body's signals and try to use the tooth right away, you'll aggravate it again and repeat the cycle. Sleep has a similar effect—by allowing your body to heal itself overnight, you prevent your inflammatory response from going into overdrive, which can prolong periods of pain. The next time you're injured, listen to your body and take some time off.

327 Try the happy diet

IF YOU'RE FEELING DOWN, EAT more omega-3 fatty acids: the same nutrients that are being touted as a preventative against major health problems including heart disease, cognitive decline, and stroke appear to help boost mood, too. New studies show that the fish-, dairy-, egg-, and flax seed–derived fat (to name a few sources) has a mitigating effect on feelings of depression. In fact, according to research from Canada, taking an omega-3 supplement helped patients with depression just as well as taking commonly prescribed medications did.

328

A spoonful of honey brings cold relief

THE NEXT TIME A BAD COUGH has you tossing and turning all night, bypass your medicine cabinet and head straight to the kitchen shelves: a number of recent studies from around the world have documented the effects of honey as a cough suppressant, and the sticky sweetener appears to work as well as, if not better than, over-the-counter cold remedies. Just ½ teaspoon of honey is more effective at reducing cough frequency than drugstore variety cough suppressants. Like cough drops, honey coats and soothes the throat, causing the cough reflex to become less active. Also, honey is antimicrobial, which means it kills germs upon contact, helping your body to fight off infection. Researchers from The Pennsylvania State University say the darker the honey, the better—browner varieties have more antioxidants than golden ones.

329

Power your workout with playlists

YOU COULD USE YOUR TIME ON the treadmill to listen to your own thoughts, but if you'd rather crank up the tunes, go for it. According to a number of studies, working out to music can help you exercise longer and harder and, best of all, sweating to your favorite songs will actually help you to enjoy exercise more too. Research has found pluses for exercising at any tempo, so just put together a playlist of songs that you know will get you moving. But be sure you change it up before you get bored, because that feeling may rub off on your workout.

330 A little waist leads to lifelong health

CALL IT MUFFIN TOP, CALL IT A beer belly. Whatever you name it, a pudgy belly can harm more than your silhouette. Scientists in Sweden found that women with low waist-to-hip ratios were 50 percent less likely to develop dementia than their bigger-bellied counterparts, and researchers suspect men would fare the same. Overall body mass didn't factor into who developed dementia—just the amount of belly fat— though it's still unclear why this centrally located flab causes so much harm to the body and mind. These findings reinforce the idea that weight around the middle is particularly harmful: other studies have linked a rounder tummy to an increased risk of heart disease and type 2 diabetes. The best way to shrink your belly is by swapping high-fat and processed foods for more vegetables, fruits, and whole grains, and by adding exercise— particularly heart-pumping, calorie-burning activities—to your daily routine.

331

Pick your fights wisely

YOU PROBABLY GRAPPLE WITH at least a few grievances each day—from kids who don't clean up their dishes after dinner to a boss who keeps taking credit for your ideas. So how do you know when to speak up and when to let it go? "Picking your battles is partly about having the wisdom to recognize when something challenges what you stand for, your basic principles," says Robert Gould, PhD, chair of the department of conflict resolution at Portland State University. In other words, if you're met with a decision or problem that's annoying, but doesn't necessarily question your system of beliefs, you might be best trying to shrug it off. But if you have a real moral dilemma on your hands—big or small—go ahead and confront it, albeit in a calm, open, and non-blaming way.

332

Shed pounds by paying attention to your sleep

SLEEP ISN'T THE CORNERSTONE of most diets, but maybe it should be. In one recent study from the University of Chicago, scientists found that people who got an adequate night's sleep while dieting lost more than twice the amount of fat than they did when they only allowed for five hours a night. In the study, the dieters' sleep time was monitored in two fourteen-day chunks: one in which they slept for a little more than seven hours each night, and one in which they were woken two hours earlier. For all four weeks, the participants ate the same number of calories and per-formed the same types of activity. Each two-week span resulted in an average loss of six pounds, but during the longer sleep-ing segments, three of those pounds were fat while only one pound of fat was shed during the two weeks of shorter rest. And, people reported being more hungry dur-ing the shorter sleep portion of the study, which supports other research showing a connection between lack of sleep and overeating.

333

Be less flaky with fitness

IF YOU'RE GOOD AT REGULATING yourself, from following through on projects to making healthy choices, you have a lot of what psychologists call "self-efficacy." But don't despair if you struggle with this—increasing your overall discipline might be as easy as starting a simple exercise routine. According to research from Jim Annesi, PhD, director of wellness advancement at the YMCA of Metropolitan Atlanta, the self-efficacy that comes from sticking with a fitness program can help you to make other positive changes in your life, like eating better. Actively committing to your health can boost your self-esteem, which makes it easier for you to make other good choices. To get started, create a reasonable fitness routine, like aiming to exercise thirty minutes a day three times a week. As you meet your fitness goals and set new ones—like increasing your activity to the recommended five days a week of exercise—you'll find that you're better able to keep on track in other areas of your life, too.

334 Positive mantras double the benefits of exercise

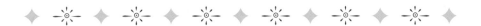

IF LOOKING IN THE MIRROR AND saying "I like myself" five times each morning seems a bit too Stuart Smalley-esque to you, it might be time to get over your self-consciousness. Research suggests that positive self-talk really does have an encouraging effect on your emotional and mental state, says Wendy Suzuki, PhD, a neuroscientist and instructor in the Center for Neural Science at New York University. For example, one recent study found that positive self-talk reduced symptoms of depression and negative thoughts in women while enhancing their self-esteem.

"There is evidence that strategies that employ positive self-affirmations to reduce negative thinking can positively impact mood and self-esteem," explains Suzuki, who also teaches intenSati, a form of cardiovascular dance that uses positive affirmations to motivate and inspire exercisers. Suzuki is still testing the effects of intenSati, but it makes perfect sense that combining positive affirmations with another mood-enhancing activity—exercise—could take your self-confidence up a notch. This idea, of course, applies outside the intenSati studio. Whatever your workout of choice, repeat a few positive phrases to yourself during each bout of fitness to feel twice as good.

335

Exercise as anti-diabetes medicine

FOR DIABETES PREVENTION YEAR after year, diet and exercise beat out the benefits of a common anti-diabetes medication, according to new findings. After a three-year U.K.-based study—and during a follow-up seven years later—overweight pre-diabetic individuals who stuck with regular exercise and a weight-reducing diet continued to have a significantly lower risk of developing type 2 diabetes than people who took medication for the condition. If your doctor reaches for the prescription pad over concerns about diabetes, bring up exercise and diet options instead. Other research has shown that losing just 7 percent of your body weight is often enough to keep you diabetes-free.

336 Let go of grudges for your health

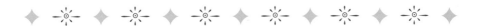

DO YOU HOLD GRUDGES, OR ARE you quick to forgive those who have wronged you? If you don't easily let go of slights and oversights, you're doing yourself a disservice: being forgiving is actually good for your health, according to Jennifer Friedberg, PhD, associate professor at New York University's School of Medicine.

In her research, Friedberg looked at people's general tendencies toward forgiveness, and how that related to overall health and blood pressure response. "Our research found that people who are more forgiving had lower cholesterol and blood pressure levels compared to people who are less forgiving," says Friedberg. "And, the people who held fewer grudges were also more likely to have their blood pressure return to normal after a stressful situation, which has been found to be a predictor of better future cardiac health." Friedberg believes this might be because forgiveness serves as a buffer against stress, depression, and anxiety, all of which can take a toll on health. Also, forgiveness promotes strong social relationships, which are associated with many positive health effects.

337 Expect the best to perform at your peak

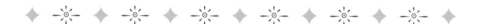

IF YOU'VE GOT A DAUNTING task ahead of you, don't waste your time worrying about how hard it's going to be. Instead, focus on how well you're going to do. According to Ayelet Fishbach, PhD, professor of behavioral science and marketing at the University of Chicago Booth School of Business, if you expect the best outcome in any possible scenario, you'll be less discouraged by obstacles than if you anticipate failure. Your optimistic attitude will help you work harder to push through challenges, resulting in greater success.

"When facing obstacles, people who are more optimistic tend to fare better," says Fishbach. For example, students who expect a test to be difficult but give themselves a pep talk beforehand perform better than those who are convinced they'll fail. By recognizing the difficulty ahead of you—and your ability to face it—you talk yourself into being able to achieve the best possible results. Of course, try to be realistic—if your hope is too great for the challenge at hand, reality may dash your optimism, leading to more negative thoughts and results.

338 To ease anxiety, listen to the sound of silence

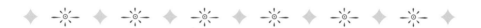

NEGATIVE MENTAL CHATTER—those little voices in your head—can lead to self-doubt, anxiety, and even depression. You may think the answer is to simply shut off those thoughts, but according to Konrad Ryushin Marchaj, abbot of the Zen Mountain Monastery and a Zen Buddhist monk, "thoughts are not the problem. It's our relationship with those thoughts that becomes problematic."

When you feel overwhelmed by negative thoughts or self-talk, don't try to distract yourself with an activity—that will only mask the problem. Instead, sit back and listen. "Mental chatter fades if you systematically engage in silence," says Marchaj.

It's natural to not want to be alone with these thoughts. But you'll find that the more you listen, the less you'll be affected. Marchaj suggests setting aside a brief period of time, such as ten minutes each morning and night, to sit in silence. As you sit, pay attention to the thoughts that come in and out of your mind but try not to dwell on them—let them slide in and out at will. Commit to this practice for two weeks, then re-evaluate at the end. If you're feeling a benefit, gradually increase the time you spend in silence.

339 Banish regret by buying what you really want

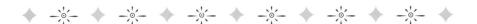

STUDIES SHOW THAT A MISSED opportunity to make a purchase—like when the store is sold out of a detergent that's on sale—will make you less likely to buy that product in the future. But then why do you still long for that jacket, painting, or other lost treasure you could have bought, but decided to forgo? According to Vanessa M. Patrick, PhD, associate professor at the University of Houston's C.T. Bauer College of Business, certain circumstances provoke this contradictory reaction, making us desire something *more*, not less, after missing a chance to buy it.

Patrick's research has found that if a purchase is tied to a goal of yours, or the item is rare, you could regret your inaction so much that you make great efforts to get the item that you once passed up. For example, if a certain one-of-a-kind rug will complete your living room, but you waffle for too long and return to the store after it's been sold, you may find yourself plotting ways to track it down. Of course, most people can't buy everything they want, but take a few moments to ask yourself how much you'll regret not purchasing an item before walking away from it, particularly if it's something that's hard to find or unique.

340 Choose flowers for foolproof gifting

THE NEXT TIME YOU'RE deliberating on the right gift to bring a friend, visit your local florist or head out to your yard with some gardening shears. According to recent research, flowers are a surefire way to get a smile.

In her research on people's reactions to flowers, Jeannette Haviland-Jones, PhD, professor of psychology at Rutgers University, recruited a group of people to participate in a mood study in her lab. But the real research began after the mood study "ended" and everyone went home: scientists, disguised as messengers, then delivered a thank-you gift to each participant in the study—either a fruit basket, a decorative candle, or a bouquet of flowers. All three gifts were well received, but only the flowers brought a smile to every single recipient's face.

341 A youthful body equals a youthful mind

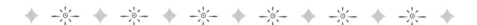

TURNS OUT THAT THE OLD adage, "You're only as old as you feel," applies not just to the body, but also to the mind. Thinking of yourself as youthful actually helps your mind stay young. That's the finding of a recent study from Purdue University in which researchers looked at the differences in "feel age" versus "real age."

In a study of nearly five hundred middle-aged people over a period of ten years, researchers found that most participants reported feeling about twelve years younger than they actually were at the start of the study. A decade later, these same people were more confident in their cognitive abilities. Conversely, those who reported feeling their actual age or older had more concern about memory loss and the other effects of aging.

While there's no single way to trick your mind and body into feeling younger, keeping up with technology and pop culture can help. So can learning new skills—studies show that both physical and mental challenges can stimulate brain growth.

342 Make teatime a daily ritual

A STEAMING CUP OF TEA CAN help you to unwind after a long day, and new research shows that some teas help you sip your way to better health, too. "A growing body of evidence suggests that consuming at least a few cups of black tea daily may reduce the risk of developing cardiovascular disease, while green teas may reduce the risk of certain cancers," says Diane L. McKay, PhD, a scientist at Tufts University's Antioxidants Research Laboratory. White teas and even herbal teas appear to have health-boosting benefits, too, and all forms of the beverage count toward your daily fluid needs and contain zero calories unless you add sugar, honey, or milk. Scientists don't yet know the exact dose of tea required to benefit health, so McKay suggests simply drinking tea regularly—a cup or three each day.

343

Eat fewer calories and have more energy

FOODS THAT HAVE A LOT OF calories can give you the fuel you need for an endurance event, like a long afternoon of cross-country skiing, but on a more typical day, these foods can actually slow you down. Calorie-dense foods require your body to work overtime, zapping your energy and leaving you sluggish. Over the long haul, eating too many energy-rich items, like meats, dairy, and highly refined foods, can lead to weight gain, says Joan Sabaté, MD, DrPH, chair and professor of nutrition at Loma Linda University's School of Public Health.

Foods like fruits, vegetables, whole grains, and legumes are nutrient-packed, lower in calories, and more energizing, says Sabaté, and they can also help with weight loss. For best health results, reach for minimally processed plant foods, suggests Sabaté. You'll get the weight-loss results you want, and feel more alive and awake after eating.

344

Phone home for a feel-good fix

DON'T BE EMBARRASSED IF THE first person you want to talk to after a bad day is your mom—it's natural. According to researchers from the University of Wisconsin-Madison, a mother's voice has confirmed soothing effects. In one recent study, scientists put girls aged seven to twelve through a nerve-rattling test, asking them to make a presentation before strangers and answer math problems. Afterward, the girls were either comforted by their mothers in person or over the phone, or they were asked to watch an emotion-free seventy-five-minute video. For the girls who were able to hug their moms or hear reassuring words over the phone, comfort quickly set in, lowering stress levels and increasing their levels of oxytocin, a hormone associated with bonding; those who watched the video didn't experience the same stress-reducing benefits. While a mother's calming effect has been largely assumed to be caused by physical contact, this study showed that simply hearing her soothing voice is enough to put you at ease.

345

Volunteer for more vim and vigor

IF YOU'VE EVER DONE VOLUNTEER work—dishing meals at a soup kitchen, walking dogs at a shelter, or reading to residents of a nursing home, for example—you probably noticed that you're full of good cheer when you leave. A number of studies back up this feeling, showing that helping others can lift symptoms of depression and improve overall life satisfaction. But the benefits don't end there: when scientists at a Finnish university analyzed the results of sixteen studies, they found that people who performed volunteer work also reported better health and higher levels of physical activity. And, in an unrelated study, researchers at Columbia University's Mailman School of Public Health found that women who were sixty-five and older and volunteered—in this case, mentoring public school children— were able to delay or even reverse cognitive decline, actually improving brain function. You're never too young or old to start volunteering: seek out a particular cause that speaks to you, and find a way to use your time and energy to benefit others.

346

Kick tummy troubles with a different coffee blend

IF YOU OFTEN SUFFER FROM AN upset stomach mid-morning, your coffee may be to blame. Coffee, which is already extremely acidic, can cause your stomach to secrete extra acid, which can lead to tummy troubles. Surprisingly, simply switching to darker coffee beans can help. According to research from the University of Vienna, lighter roasts tend to irritate the stomach more than darker roasts. Researchers think that a longer roasting process causes these positive effects—steamed or lightly roasted beans appear to aggravate the stomach more—but the results may also be due to the dark bean's lower caffeine content. Whatever the reason, the results are in: the next time you order coffee or buy your own beans, the darker the better.

347 See yourself in how you see others

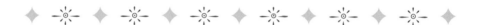

IF YOU TEND TO SEE THE BEST IN people, you're more than just an optimist: how we view the world and those in it is a clear indication of how we see ourselves. "Our perceptions of others can tell us a lot about ourselves," says Simine Vazire, PhD, assistant professor of psychology at Washington University in St. Louis.

According to Vazire, our judgments reflect back on ourselves. For example, if you're agreeable and happy, you'll likely judge a new person in a positive light. According to Vazire's research, the more positively you rate others, the more likely you'll be judged as agreeable, conscientious, and emotionally stable.

Of course, the opposite is also true: if you're negative or disagreeable, whether it's conscious or not, you may see others in a less positive light, and that may affect the impression you leave, too. Moral of the story: the next time you meet someone new, pay attention to how you perceive them—it may say something about you.

348

Practice volume control for healthy hearing

YOU MAY WEAR HEADPHONES to listen to tunes while you exercise or commute. But if you have to adjust the volume of your music to hear a question someone asks you, your headphones may be damaging your hearing. That's the latest from scientists at Pace University in New York. The large-scale study tracked the hearing of more than eight thousand girls over a period of twenty-four years. The number of study participants who used handheld music players like iPods quadrupled between 2001 and 2008; over that same period, hearing loss rose by 7 percent, and the occurrence of ringing of the ears and other hearing problems rose by 8 percent. Scientists cannot say for certain that the headphones were the cause, but to keep your hearing in good condition, adjust your headphone volume so that you're able to hear a nearby person speak.

349 Wake up your body with morning moves

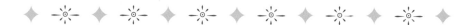

TO WAKE UP YOUR MIND IN THE morning, you may sip on a cup of coffee or read the day's newspaper. But what sort of ritual do you have to wake up your body? Taking a few moments to tune in to your body before getting out of bed allows you to shake off your slumber and helps you to move more efficiently throughout the day, says Alycea Ungaro, owner of Real Pilates, a fitness center in New York, and author of the *Pilates Practice Companion*.

Here is Ungaro's daily wake-up ritual: In bed, lengthen your body, reaching your arms overhead and stretching your fingers and toes away from each other. After a few breaths, tense the muscles, flexing the feet and hands, arching the back, and squeezing the legs together. Hold for a few seconds then relax, going limp. When you're ready to sit up, do so gradually. Spin so that your calves dangle off the bed, and round over your thighs. Hold for a few breaths, then slowly roll up through the spine. If your body still isn't feeling awake, do more stretching in the shower, says Ungaro, where the heat of the water will help loosen your muscles.

350 Ease your anxiety about anxiety

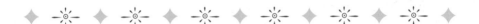

ANXIETY CAN BE DEBILITATING. In addition to a racing mind, it's often accompanied by a pounding heart, feelings of being out of control, and even numbness. It's these symptoms, and the fear they inspire, that make anxiety worse, says Michael Otto, PhD, professor of psychology at Boston University and co-author of *Living with Bipolar Disorder: A Guide for Individuals and Families.*

It may seem counterintuitive, but the best way to treat anxiety is simply to accept it. "Getting comfortable with your anxiety is extremely beneficial," says Otto. While anxiety is unpleasant, going to lengths to avoid the situations that prompt it will only make the anxiety worse. If you start changing your behavior and habits, you're letting your fears take over and increasing the chance that future bouts of anxiety will only be more severe. Instead, when anxious feelings arise, pause for a moment to take inventory of what is happening. "When you're familiar with the signals of anxiety—if you acknowledge it's happening and know why—you'll have a more comfortable state reaction, which means you're better able to deal," says Otto. Your anxiety will likely last for less time, and will gradually happen less often.

351

Cure malaise over mealtime

ACCORDING TO AYURVEDIC tradition, good health comes from a strong fire in the belly. Many different things can snuff out the flame, says Ayurvedic medicine teacher Laura Plumb, including eating too much food, or consuming food that is processed, heavy, or old. If your general state of mind is anything but light, clear, peaceful, or stable, or if you're feeling sluggish, a low-burning fire may be to blame.

"If you're feeling heavy, bloated, lethargic, or cloudy-headed, try fasting by skipping dinner one night each week," suggests Plumb. "Or, stick to a liquid vegetable diet for a day or two, sipping warm vegetable soups and broths in lieu of meals." This sort of detox can help stoke your internal fire and bring balance back to your body and mind. According to Plumb, drinking lemon and ginger tea throughout the day and with meals will also help with digestion and flushing out toxins, and so will adding ginger to your diet.

352 Couple-up to squelch stress

HERE'S A BIT OF SCIENCE TO keep in mind the next time your partner starts to drive you crazy: being part of a pair puts you less at risk for high levels of stress. Those were the findings in a new University of Chicago study that tracked hormone levels during stressful situations. Among the single people, levels of cortisol—the stress hormone—skyrocketed, while couples in romantic partnerships (married or not) experienced milder peaks. Scientists believe this is another indication that social support can buffer the effects of stress, a theory that has been proven in other types of relationships, such as among friends and family.

353 Don't give away all the answers

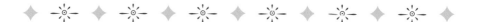

WHEN A FRIEND ASKS YOU TO help her make a difficult decision, your first instinct may be to weigh the odds, then tell her what you think she should do. And, while this sequence may feel natural and easy, an answer to her problem is probably not what your friend needs, says Parker Palmer, PhD, author of *A Hidden Wholeness: The Journey Toward an Undivided Life* and founder of the Center for Courage and Renewal, an organization devoted to helping people to bring positive change to their lives.

"One of my favorite definitions of love is the willingness to extend yourself for the benefit of another person's growth," says Palmer. "But even though a lot of what we do for love is well-intended, it's also self serving." When it comes to giving guidance, stepping back is often the only way to help a person grow, even if she'd prefer you just tell her what to do. "If you're a good teacher, you need to be willing to say I'm not going to give you the answer, because I wouldn't be teaching you if I did." To help someone discover her own solutions, ask open-ended questions to encourage her to clarify what her thoughts really are.

354 Make plans when you're feeling positive

IF YOU'RE FEELING DISCONTENT with your present circumstances, it may seem like the perfect time to plan for your future, because you've got real incentive to move forward. But according to Vanessa M. Patrick, PhD, associate professor at the University of Houston's C.T. Bauer College of Business, when you're unhappy, you have a harder time forming abstract thoughts—like the big picture of your life—and instead slip back into worrying about more immediate concerns, like that overwhelming work project. As tempting as it may be to start daydreaming about things to come, put off goal-setting and future-planning until you're feeling upbeat and hopeful again, suggests Patrick. This will ensure that you're better able to focus on your long-term goals and vision of your future. Or, take action to change your frame of mind: Patrick recommends reminiscing or writing about one of the happiest days of your life, or looking over a list of ten positive words to make over your mood in an instant.

355 Speak the language of support

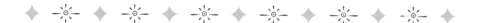

IF YOU'VE EVER GONE THROUGH a tough time (and who hasn't), you know just how important it is to have the support of close ones. Science backs up this shoulder-to-cry-on theory: In a recent study, psychologists correctly predicted the likelihood of recovery in heart failure patients simply by assessing the relationship between the patient and his or her spouse. The stronger the bond, the more likely the patient's health would improve over the next six months.

Interestingly, the couple's own assessment of the strength of their marriage wasn't the most accurate measure of the relationship's ability to heal. Rather, the most telling results were found when researchers analyzed how frequently the patients' spouses used "we" versus "I" when describing how they had coped with the recent health problems of their partners. The ones whose spouses used "we" more often had a higher chance of recovery.

Why is swapping "I" for "we" so powerful? "'We-talk' suggests that the speakers view the situation in a broader, more inclusive way, and that can lead to feelings of social inclusion, belonging, or support," says Matthias R. Mehl, PhD, assistant professor in the University of Arizona's department of psychology, and co-author of the study. While the speaker may say "we" simply out of habit, it indicates—probably subconsciously—that the patient is not going through the ordeal alone.

356 Nourish your soul with creative time

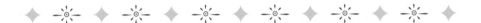

IT MAY SEEM SELF-INDULGENT OR unimportant to make time for the creative pursuits you enjoy, like an afternoon to write or draw, or a weekend to immerse yourself in dance and song. But the benefits often outweigh the time cost, says James Kullander, program curriculum developer at the Omega Institute for Holistic Studies, a retreat center with a mind-body focus in New York state, and a writer who has taught workshops on writing as meditation.

"When you engage in a creative pastime, that to-do list you carry with you becomes less important," says Kullander. "Your true source of creativity resides in the deep wellspring of your soul. By tapping this, you'll be better equipped to lead a happy, meaningful life,

and you'll keep yourself more alive." And, as you nourish your own needs, you'll become more in tune with the needs of those around you, too.

If your favorite activities aren't traditional arts like writing or painting or making music, they can still bring the same benefits if you approach them with passion. "Cooking is an act of creativity, and so is raising children," says Kullander. "Our entire life is an ongoing act of creation." Whatever moves you to drop your worries, abandon your checklist, and work with zest toward a greater good—from enrolling in piano lessons to forming an organization to improve your local grade school—is worth pursuing for the balance it can bring to your life.

357

Sweat can help you sleep

NEED SOME SHUT-EYE? TRY adding aerobic activity to your schedule. A new study from Northwestern University's Feinberg School of Medicine found that insomniacs who did just 160 minutes of cardio each week slept better. Interestingly, when compared to another study on the effects of the slow movements of Tai Chi on sleep, aerobic exercise rated tops at prompting extra Zs. Scientists are unsure what exactly about aerobic activity brings on better sleep, but if you're having a hard time dozing off, hit the gym before you hit the hay. Even a late-night sweat session will do: recent research shows that exercising right before bedtime doesn't make it harder for most people to fall asleep.

358 Healthy behaviors add up

MOST SCIENTIFIC STUDIES FOCUS on single subjects—for instance, the value of eating healthful foods or engaging in regular aerobic activity. Few studies look at how combining several healthy behaviors can maximize our well-being. But a recent large-scale review of the health of more than seventy-thousand Chinese women by Vanderbilt University does just that.

In the report, which gathered data from the Shanghai Women's Health Study, non-smoking and non-drinking women aged forty to seventy were given one point for each of five healthy behaviors they engaged in: staying at a normal weight, having a low level of belly fat, regularly exercising, having little exposure to second-hand cigarette smoke, and maintaining a higher than average fruit and vegetable intake. Those who accumulated four or five points were about half as likely to pass away from any cause during the nine-year study as those who scored zero.

359 Make your yoga fit your mood

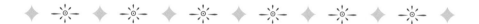

DO YOU TURN TO YOGA TO GAIN energy, or move through the poses as a way to relax? Chances are, you look for different outcomes depending on your mood and the time of day; luckily, all it takes is a few adjustments to your practice to get your desired result. Small changes to yoga sequences can affect your mind and body in different ways, says Ayurvedic medicine teacher and yoga instructor Laura Plumb, cofounder of the Deep Yoga School of Healing Arts in San Diego. During the day, when you want to feel alert, aim to increase your circulation by moving quickly through a sequence that has many standing poses, says Plumb. If you're practicing at night, or at a time when you want to unwind, your goal should be to calm the body and mind, says Plumb. Modify challenging poses to make them easier, move more slowly, and add more seated and lying down poses to your practice. Change your breath and intention to fit your goal, too: To get a lift, use deep, powerful breaths and be tuned in to your environment. To unwind, turn your focus inward and pause throughout the practice; by holding poses for longer periods, you'll be able to slow the breath and the mind.

360 Stop loneliness before it spreads

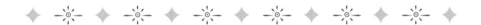

IF YOU'VE EVER FELT LONELY, even with other people around, you're not, well, alone. Feelings of connectedness vary from person to person, and can change quickly. "You can feel very lonely even though you're surrounded by people, or you can feel completely content when you're alone," says James Fowler, PhD, professor at the University of California, San Diego, and co-author of *Connected: The Surprising Power of Our Social Networks and How They Shape Our Lives*. And, just as laughter can pass from person to person, loneliness, too, can spread throughout a social network.

Fowler recently performed a study of this idea of loneliness within a group in an effort to understand ways to stop its spread. "People with fewer friends tend to feel more lonely, but they're still not alone," says Fowler. However, the symptoms of depression and negativity that often come with loneliness can influence a person's network, causing those close to them to withdraw—breaking the connection—or to take on some of the negativity, either of which can bring more feelings of loneliness.

"On the edge of the networks, there's a fraying, so if you pull on the thread, it can unravel," explains Fowler. But you can stop the unraveling of a network: When you protect the people on the periphery—those who are likely to be the loneliest—you'll protect the network. So when you notice someone in your circle is going through a rough time, reach out and offer support. This way you'll ease his or her loneliness and stop feelings of isolation from spreading.

361

Lower your blood pressure with fitness blasts

BATTLING HYPERTENSION DOESN'T need to take several months and a pile of prescriptions—a pair of sneakers might be all you need. Brazilian researchers recently found that short spurts of moderate-intensity exercise can lower blood pressure as effectively as commonly prescribed medications can. In the study, just twenty minutes of running on a treadmill or circuit training was enough to lower blood pressure for more than seven hours, including time spent at work, when stress levels—and blood pressure—tend to spike. Before ditching your meds cold turkey, talk to your doctor about creating a plan for easing into an exercise-based treatment. If you opt for weight lifting, perform rapid sets: it's unclear if the positive results from the circuit training were due to gains in strength or the cardiovascular aspect of the exercise.

362 Sing a song to lose the blues

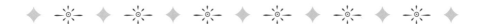

YOU MAY NOT WIN A GRAMMY anytime soon—or even get up the guts to hop onstage at your local karaoke bar—but that's no reason not to belt out the occasional tune on your own time. The simple act of breaking out in song has been shown to lift your spirits, says Ann Skingley, PhD, senior researcher at the Sidney De Haan Research Centre for Arts and Health at Canterbury Christ Church University in New Zealand.

"In our interviews with older people who took part in group singing, an uplifting effect on mood was certainly apparent," says Skingley. In fact, according to her work, singing may be even more effective at making people happy than listening to music is, because it requires active participation. Whether you sing your heart out in the shower or join a local choir, you'll increase positive feelings by making more opportunities to use your voice as an instrument. According to Skingley, the benefits of song extend beyond the psychological, with research indicating that singing may ease some chronic conditions, reducing anger in dementia sufferers or aiding in breath control for people with pulmonary disease.

363 Stretch for your health

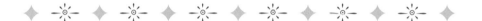

BEING FLEXIBLE REDUCES MUSCLE pulls and injuries during exercise, and studies have also shown that stretching decreases soreness after a tough workout. Keeping the joints open and mobile is important for everyday activities, too: stretching helps us maintain our range of motion, which tends to decrease with age, says Kristin McGee, a yoga and Pilates instructor in New York City.

It's best to stretch the muscles when they're warm, says McGee, so add five to ten minutes of flexibility work to the end of a workout, or do a brief warm-up before stretching, such as jumping jacks or marching in place. Ease into each stretch, and don't push yourself too hard. "Once you feel a slight pull, ease off slightly and hold where you are for a few breaths, then try to go a bit further," recommends McGee. Stretch the muscles you tend to use most, such as the fronts and backs of the thighs and the chest, staying in each stretch for thirty to sixty seconds. Stretch at least a few times a week to see gains in flexibility.

364

Solidify friendships with small gestures

IF YOU WANT TO MAKE A FRIEND for life, one thoughtful gesture may be all it takes. At least those were the findings in one recent study from the University of Virginia. In the study, sorority sisters were asked to give anonymous gifts to pledges; regardless of gift size or cost, the presents that recipients felt were the most thoughtful—that most catered to their specific likes and interests—inspired the greatest bonds between the recipient and the gift giver. While home-baked goodies are sure to win favor with anyone, more personalized acts of kindness—such as an offer to read an acquaintance's cover letter or gifting a small trinket that reminds you of a fun time with a friend—may mean more. Whatever the gift, keep it within a reasonable budget— people may feel the need to reciprocate large tokens of affection, which can cancel out the good feelings.

365 Aim to resolve an argument, not just win it

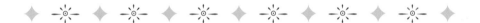

PICTURE THE LAST TIME YOU GOT into a disagreement: When you weren't the one talking, were you listening to the other person and trying to see his or her point of view, or were you distracted, trying to formulate your next statement of opposition? "A common mistake people make during a conflict is listening only long enough to hear a point they disagree with so they can then pounce on that point with their own argument," says Lynne Hurdle-Price, president of Hurdle-Price Professionals, a conflict resolution and diversity awareness consulting organization. But that's not the best tactic if you want a resolution.

"One of the best techniques in conflict resolution is to give the gift of listening to the other person," says Hurdle-Price. "Use active listening and open questions to find out as much as possible about what their thoughts, feelings, and issues are before you state your own position." This will allow the other person to feel heard, which will help de-escalate emotions and can help you to build a clearer list of specific issues to address.

Acknowledgments

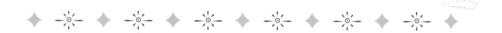

THIS BOOK COULD NOT HAVE been written without the generosity of the nearly two hundred experts who believed in the project and contributed their time and thoughts to make it a success. I learned so much, and will be forever thankful for the way these 365 suggestions have changed my life. Closer to home, I'm indebted to my friend Alyssa Way, who helped light the spark behind *Better Each Day* over a beer at La Guardia airport—I'm so glad our flight was delayed that day! My agent, Mollie Glick, was a champion of this project from the start—her keen sense really helped me define the scope of the book. Thanks to my lovely editor, Jodi Warshaw, for being kind in her notes and for embracing my vision. I'm also grateful for the tutelage and guidance the *Prevention* magazine staff has provided me, particularly Michele Stanten, Margot Gilman, Robbie Caploe, and, of course, Diane Salvatore. My parents, Michael and Connie Cassity, offered encouragement and support from start to finish—thank you for instilling in me the drive and determination to see this project through. Finally, thanks to my mutual appreciation society: Rebecca Cassity, Lisa Galaites, Christie Anderson, Evelyn Spence, and the girls of 275, who kept me inspired and amused when the days—though better—also grew long.

Index

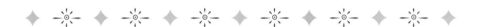

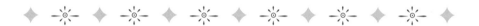